Research Ethics

Medicine in the twenty-first century is increasingly reliant on research to guarantee the safety and efficacy of medical interventions. As a result, it is essential to understand the ethical issues that research generates. This volume introduces the principal areas of concern in research on human subjects, offering a framework for understanding research ethics, and the relationship between ethics and compliance.

Research Ethics brings together leading scholars in bioethics and the topics covered include the unique concerns that arise in specific areas of research such as gene therapy and stem cell research. Individual chapters also address the ethical issues that arise when conducting research with specific populations such as infants, children, or adolescents, and the volume looks at important emerging issues in human subjects research, namely financial conflicts of interest and the interpretation of scientific data.

Ana Smith Iltis teaches health-care ethics at Saint Louis University in St. Louis, Missouri, USA and her research interests are human subjects research ethics and organizational ethics.

Routledge Annals of Bioethics

Series editors:

Mark J. Cherry
Saint Edwards University, USA

Ana Smith Iltis
Saint Louis University, USA

Bioethics has become a truly international phenomenon. Secular Western bioethics in particular lays claim to a universal account of proper moral deportment, including the foundations of law and public policy as well as the moral authority for national and international institutions to guarantee uniformity of practice, secure basic human rights, and promote social justice.

Through foundational, philosophical, religious, and cultural perspectives, clinical case studies, and legal analyses, the books in this series document, review, and explore emerging bioethical viewpoints as well as the state of the art of this global endeavor. Volumes will critically appreciate diverse legal, moral, cultural, and religious viewpoints representing the various regions of the world, from mainland China and Hong Kong, Taiwan, Japan, India, and East Asia more generally, to Europe, the Middle East, Australia, and New Zealand, to South America and North America. Moral perspectives range from Orthodox Christianity, Roman Catholicism, and contemporary Protestant Christianity, to Orthodox, Conservative, and Reformed Judaism, to Islam, Buddhism, Confucianism, Hinduism, and so forth, to secular liberalism.

The Annals of Bioethics compasses monographs and edited volumes on moral theory, normative health-care practice, case studies, and public policy as well as volumes documenting and assessing legal, religious, and cultural responses to specific aspects of the fast-paced developments in health care and medical technology.

1   **Research Ethics**
    Edited by Ana Smith Iltis

Previous titles to appear in the Routledge Annals of Bioethics include:

Regional Perspectives in Bioethics
Edited by Mark J. Cherry and John F. Peppin

Religious Perspectives on Bioethics
Edited by Mark J. Cherry, Ana Iltis, and John F. Peppin

Research Ethics

Edited by
Ana Smith Iltis

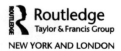

Routledge
Taylor & Francis Group

NEW YORK AND LONDON

First published 2006
by Routledge
270 Madison Ave, New York, NY 10016

Simultaneously published in the UK
by Routledge
2 Park Square, Milton Park, Abingdon, Oxon OX14 4RN

Routledge is an imprint of the Taylor & Francis Group

Typeset in Garamond by
Newgen Imaging Systems (P) Ltd, Chennai, India
Printed and bound in Great Britain by
Biddles Ltd, King's Lynn

Library of Congress Cataloging in Publication Data
A catalog record for this book has been requested

British Library Cataloguing in Publication Data
A catalogue record for this book is available from the British Library

ISBN 0–415–70158–9

Contents

Tables

Contributors

Lauren Matukaitis Broyles, BSN, BA, RN, Predoctoral Fellow, School of Nursing and Center for Bioethics and Health Law, University of Pittsburgh, Pittsburgh, Pennsylvania.

Mark J. Cherry, PhD, Associate Professor, Department of Philosophy, Saint Edward's University, Austin, Texas.

James M. DuBois, PhD, DSc, Associate Professor, PhD Program Director, Center for Health Care Ethics, Saint Louis University, St. Louis, Missouri.

Christine Grady, RN, PhD, FAAN, Head, Section on Human Subjects Research, Department of Clinical Bioethics, W.G. Magnuson Clinical Center, National Institutes of Health, Bethesda, Maryland.

Ana Smith Iltis, PhD, Assistant Professor, Center for Health Care Ethics, Saint Louis University, St. Louis, Missouri.

Loretta M. Kopelman, PhD, Chair, Department of Medical Humanities, Brody School of Medicine, East Carolina University, Greenville, North Carolina.

Gerard Magill, PhD, Professor, Executive Director, Department Chair, Center for Health Care Ethics, Saint Louis University, St. Louis, Missouri.

Lisa S. Parker, PhD, Associate Professor of Human Genetics, Director of Graduate Education, Center for Bioethics and Health Law, University of Pittsburgh, Pittsburgh, Pennsylvania.

David B. Resnik, JD, PhD, Department of Medical Humanities, Brody School of Medicine, East Carolina University, Greenville, North Carolina. Current affiliation: Bioethicist, National Institutes of Environmental Health Services/National Institutes of Health, Research Triangle Park, North Carolina.

Griffin Trotter, MD, PhD, Associate Professor, Center for Health Care Ethics, Saint Louis University, St. Louis, Missouri.

Acknowledgments

I would like to express my gratitude to the Center for Health Care Ethics, the Graduate School, and my colleagues at Saint Louis University for their ongoing support of this and other endeavors. I owe a special debt of gratitude to Barbara Anne Hinze, who spent countless hours editing and formatting this volume.

Ana Smith Iltis
Saint Louis University

1 Human subjects research

Ethics and compliance

Ana Smith Iltis

Medicine in the twenty-first century will be defined by biomedical research. Research is not merely experimentation but any systematic assessment of interventions aimed at making public the results.[1] Because of the need for outcomes research to confirm the safety and efficacy of medical interventions, health care is increasingly coming to have a research component. We have become acutely aware of an epistemological problem in medicine: it is very difficult to know that we know truly, and thus the history of medicine is riddled with fads. At one time, we accepted that ulcers should be treated with rest and dietary changes rather than antibiotics, which we later learned were necessary to fight the bacteria *Helicobacter pylori* that cause ulcers (Cherry 2002). Similarly, it was accepted that premature infants should be exposed to high concentrations of oxygen, which we later learned led to blindness (Cohen 1998). These are only examples of cases in which a certain approach to treating a condition became a standard of care without the systematic assessment of outcomes. Once outcomes were measured, the error in judgment was clear. The medical community has learned that true knowledge is available only by measuring outcomes, that is, by engaging in research. This epistemological problem brings with it an important moral problem: it is immoral to treat patients in suboptimal ways if the opportunity exists to determine and then do, without serious burden, what is best. This results in what we might call the research imperative: there is an obligation to assess outcomes so as to provide the best treatment possible in the future. Thus, there is a growing focus on assessing interventions in routine clinical care. Moreover, there is the drive to decrease morbidity and mortality through new technologies. We can expect that interest in biomedical research will be central to health care in the future. As such, understanding the ethical issues that research generates is increasingly important.

This volume focuses on the ethical conduct of research on human persons. This introduction identifies some of the critical episodes in the history of biomedical research that have shaped our current understanding of research ethics.[2] Special attention is given to the regulations and regulatory bodies governing biomedical research in the United States, particularly to the often-cited sections of the Code of Federal Regulations (CFR) governing research (45CFR46; 21CFR50; 21CFR56).[3] The focus on regulations governing research is not meant to imply that research ethics is equivalent to regulatory compliance. However, the regulations and guidelines discussed here largely have been written out of concern to ensure the ethical conduct of research and thus they reflect much of what are widely accepted as necessary conditions for the ethical use of humans in biomedical research. Regulations often do not capture emerging issues, and many of the contributions to the volume point to debates, concerns, dilemmas, and problems that are not resolvable merely through regulatory compliance. Nevertheless, an understanding of the regulatory climate within which research is conducted is essential to understanding the broader scope of research ethics.

Pivotal events in the history of biomedical research ethics

Much of what we take for granted today as the minimum standards for the ethical conduct of biomedical research on human persons is the result of less than 100 years of attention to human subjects research. This is not to say that prior to the twentieth century no attention had been given to the appropriate uses of humans in research. For example, in the fifteenth century, Cajetan identified the exploitation of the poor in medical experimentation as problematic (Amundsen 1981a,b). But to a large extent it was the publicity surrounding some of the events in biomedical research in the early to middle part of the twentieth century that generated concern over biomedical research and that fueled the development of standards to govern research on human persons.

During the Holocaust, Nazi physicians performed extraordinarily painful and often deadly experiments on human persons without their consent. Some of the most well-known examples are the twin studies performed in Auschwitz and Birkenau under the direction of Josef Mengele and the hypothermia experiments conducted in Dachau.[4] Details of the Nazi experiments conducted in concentration camps emerged in the Nuremberg Trials, during which twenty-three German doctors and scientists were charged with crimes against humanity for their participation in experimentation on human persons. Part of the judgment against the physicians included the development of ten principles that ought to be followed when using humans in research. These principles, known as The Nuremberg Code (1947/1949: 181–82), include the obligation (1) to obtain the voluntary consent of the persons involved as subjects; (2) to allow persons to end their participation in a study at any time; (3) to ensure that research is needed to obtain the information sought (i.e., it could not be obtained in some other way) and that the research is expected to be beneficial to society; (4) to minimize the risks to the subjects and the suffering they are likely to experience; and (5) to ensure that the expected benefits outweigh the risks. These principles have been central to many of the other documents pertaining to research ethics that have been developed since 1947.[5]

Subsequent to the Nuremberg Code, other internationally recognized guidelines for the ethical conduct of research were developed. The Declaration of Helsinki was adopted by the World Medical Association in 1964 and includes the basic principles outlined in the Nuremberg Code. The Declaration of Helsinki was revised in 1975, 1983, 1989, 1996, 2000, and a brief note regarding placebo-controlled trials was added in 2002. One of the most influential additions to the Declaration was the 1975 suggestion that research protocols be submitted for review to an independent group that could assess the research (Brody 1998: 34). This independent committee is what we know of today as the Institutional Review Board (IRB) or the Ethics Review Board (ERB).

Only two years after the Declaration of Helsinki was written, the medical community in the United States faced serious public allegations of violating the rights of research subjects. In 1966, the *New England Journal of Medicine* published an article by Henry Beecher in which he cited twenty-two biomedical studies involving human persons that were, in his opinion, unethical. Among these were the Jewish Chronic Disease Hospital study involving the injection of live liver cancer cells into elderly patients without their consent and the Willowbrook hepatitis study.[6] Between 1956 and 1972, many of the children living at the Willowbrook State School for the Retarded in New York were injected with hepatitis in order to study the possible use of gamma globulin to treat hepatitis in the early stages of infection. Staff members at the institution routinely were given gamma globulin to prevent infection. Most of the residents of Willowbrook developed hepatitis during their tenure there, and investigators thought that it would be helpful to find a way to treat them before the infection became severe. By intentionally infecting them, they knew exactly when they had developed the infection and could begin treatment promptly. This study was carried out with the approval of and funding by the Armed Forces Epidemiological Board. Consent was obtained from the children's parents, though there were allegations of coercion. There were two "tracks" for admission to the institution: one for children whose parents agreed to enroll them in the study and one for those who did not. Space for children scheduled to participate in the hepatitis study opened much more quickly than for those who were not going to participate. As a result, parents desperate to place their children in Willowbrook were much more likely to be willing to consent to their children's research participation (ACHRE 1995: chapter 3).

Prior to Beecher's publication, attention already had been given to ethical issues in biomedical research in the United States, but his article increased awareness of inappropriate actions by physicians toward persons in the name of conducting biomedical research. Other studies soon would be identified that also involved unethical practices. One of the most well-known studies was conducted by the United States Public Health Service and involved observing the natural progression of syphilis in African American sharecroppers in Alabama. When the observational study began in 1932 there was no known safe and effective treatment for syphilis. The study was designed to observe men infected with syphilis and record the progression of their disease. It was carried out without their permission or knowledge. The men were told that they would receive free medical care but were never told that they were research subjects and that there was no benefit to them for being in the study. At its inception the study was problematic because the subjects had not given their informed consent and did not know they were involved in research. As the study progressed, it became known that penicillin could be used to effectively treat the disease and penicillin became widely available in the United States. Yet subjects were not told about this, and measures were taken to discourage them from seeking treatment elsewhere. Many of these subjects suffered the consequences of untreated syphilis, including blindness and insanity. The study continued until 1973 (ACHRE 1995: chapter 3; Jones 1981).[7]

The Office for the Protection from Research Risks (OPRR) was created in 1972 under the National Institutes of Health (NIH) to protect the welfare of human research subjects. The present day Office of Human Research Protections (OHRP), housed under the Department of Health and Human Services, is a descendant of OPRR. Initially, OPRR was responsible for overseeing NIH-sponsored research that was carried out at other institutions. Today, the OHRP oversees all research in the United States that is federally funded or that is conducted in or by institutions that receive federal funding. OHRP also issues interpretive guidelines for how federal regulations governing research are to be understood and applied. (See, e.g., the *IRB Guidebook*, OHRP 2001.)

The revelations of unethical studies led the US Congress to become more interested in establishing standards to govern biomedical research and, in 1974, Congress passed the National Research Act, requiring IRB review of some research protocols. The National Commission for the Protection of Research Subjects of Biomedical and Behavioral Research also was appointed under the Act. The Commission was assigned the task of identifying principles and guidelines that ought to govern research on human persons.[8] In 1979, the Commission produced *The Belmont Report*, which identified three basic ethical principles that should govern research on human persons and described the implications of each principle for biomedical research. To a significant extent, the findings published in *The Belmont Report* continue to frame our understanding of research ethics. The three principles are:

1   Respect for Persons: The judgments of autonomous persons, those "capable of deliberation about personal goals and of acting under the direction of such deliberation," must be respected. And those who are not autonomous and thus are not capable of self-determination must be given special protections (B.1).
2   Beneficence: To treat persons ethically requires that one protect them from harm and make efforts to secure their well-being. Thus, the principle of beneficence requires that those conducting research on human persons "(1) do not harm and (2) maximize possible benefits and minimize possible harms" (B.2).
3   Justice: The principle of justice concerns the distribution of benefits and burdens in research. It requires that one avoid denying someone a benefit to which he is entitled and that one avoid imposing an undue burden on a person (B.3).

According to *The Belmont Report*, each principle generates particular requirements in the research context. The principle of respect for persons gives us the obligation to obtain subjects' informed consent. To be valid, sufficient information must be presented to subjects in a manner and context in which they can understand it. Consent must be voluntary and free from coercion (C.1). The principle of beneficence requires that the expected benefits of the research (to subjects and/or society) outweigh the risks associated with it, subjects never be treated inhumanely, risks to subjects be minimized, research involving significant risk be thoroughly assessed to ensure that the benefits outweigh the risks, special attention be given to research that will put vulnerable subjects at risk, and potential subjects be informed of the potential risks and benefits of participating in research (C.2). Finally, the principle of justice requires "that there be fair procedures and outcomes in the selection of research subjects. No one population should be unduly burdened by participation in research, nor should one population be offered the opportunity to participate in potentially beneficial research while others are denied the opportunity" (C.3).[9]

The minimum conditions that must be met to conduct research on human persons in an ethical manner established in *The Belmont Report* are embodied in the US CFR (45CFR46 and 21CFR50). The CFR provides extensive detail on the application of the principles of research ethics and establishes numerous requirements that individuals and institutions engaged in human subjects research must meet. These central elements are discussed later.

The term "Common Rule" is often used to refer to the regulations governing research in the CFR. In 1991, seventeen federal agencies and departments that participated in and had jurisdiction over human subjects research agreed to adopt common rules to govern research on human persons. The Food and Drug Administration (FDA) maintains its own set of requirements, though they overlap significantly with the Common Rule.[10]

The CFR governs only research conducted in the United States or by investigators from the United States who are engaged in research outside the United States when the research is sponsored by the US government or by institutions that receive federal funding, or when those investigators work for institutions that require them to comply with federal regulations (usually because those institutions receive federal funding and have a federal-wide assurance that binds them to conduct all human subjects research in accordance with federal regulations).[11] Privately funded research conducted by institutions that do not receive federal funding, by investigators who do not work for institutions that receive federal funding, and the results of which are not to be submitted to the FDA as part of an application for FDA approval, is not subject to the CFR. Some of the work done by private biotechnology companies, for example, is not subject to the CFR.[12] In recent years, some private companies whose research is not regulated by the CFR and who are not required to have IRBs have established their own research ethics review boards, often called Ethical Advisory Boards (EABs). These boards have been the subject of great controversy in the bioethics literature, primarily because of questions concerning the extent to which EABs can provide truly independent review and the extent to which their recommendations are or are not binding.[13]

The Council for International Organization of Medical Sciences (CIOMS) was established in 1949 by the World Health Organization (WHO) and United Nations Educational, Scientific and Cultural Organisation (UNESCO). CIOMS has developed a number of documents concerning research ethics, the most comprehensive of which appeared in 1982, 1993, and 2002. The CIOMS guidelines cover many of the same points addressed in the Nuremberg Code, the Declaration of Helsinki, *The Belmont Report*, and the CFR, including the obligation to obtain free and informed consent of human research subjects and the requirement that research protocols be reviewed by an independent committee prior to commencing research. They also address the inclusion of vulnerable groups in biomedical research, such as children and individuals with mental or behavioral disorders, and the protections that must be offered to such persons. These guidelines are not binding in the United States, but they often inform research ethics discussions and can shape our understanding and interpretation of the federal regulations governing research.

Central elements of the ethical conduct of human subjects research

The CFR sets minimum ethical standards; research cannot be considered ethical merely by meeting these minimum requirements. There are special concerns that arise in numerous areas of human subjects research that are not explicitly addressed by the CFR or on which the regulations leave room for interpretation. Some of these special concerns are addressed in this volume. This section introduces common concerns and rules that pertain to human subjects research in general. While the discussion here is grounded in the CFR and thus in research ethics as it is understood in the United States, much of what is discussed in the CFR bears significant resemblance to regulations governing research elsewhere, especially in Canada, Europe, Australia, New Zealand, and Japan.

Before research may begin, a research protocol generally must be reviewed and approved by a duly constituted IRB. The IRB must be composed of at least five persons, one of whom has a background in science and one who does not, and at least one member must not be affiliated with the institution in question. The membership should be diverse and sensitive to cultural, religious, and ethnic differences that might pertain to persons participating in research at the institution (45CFR46.107). In addition, research that involves prisoners must be reviewed by an IRB that has at least one member suited to represent the interests of the subject population. Although most research requires IRB review and approval, there are provisions for exempting certain kinds of research altogether and for expediting the review of certain types of protocols that do not require review by the full board. For example, generally, research that involves only the use of existing data when that data is recorded by investigators without identifiers or codes such that it is impossible to identify the persons whose information is being studied may be exempt (see 45CFR46.101b). Many institutions require that IRBs be notified of an investigator's intent to conduct exempt research and that the institution confirm that the proposed research is in fact exempt. Some research requires IRB review but qualifies for an expedited review, which is conducted either by the chair of the IRB or by a designated, experienced reviewer (45CFR46.110). Research that may be reviewed on an expedited basis includes protocols that involve only minimal risk to subjects and fall into one of nine categories specified by the Secretary of the Department of Health and Human Services (DHHS).[14] Examples include studies that involve only the collection of biological specimens through noninvasive measures and studies involving the collection of limited amounts of blood.

The overall goal of IRB review is to ensure that the research protocol itself meets the necessary standards established in the CFR and that the investigators plan to carry out the research in a way that protects research participants. The principal considerations of IRB review are the conditions set forth in the CFR (45CFR46.111), although individual institutions may have additional requirements. First, risks to participants must be minimized and the expected benefits of the study must outweigh the risks. Often subjects themselves do not stand to benefit from participation in research, but the knowledge that we can expect to gain through the research is significant enough that it warrants exposing individuals to a certain level of risk or burden, provided that measures are taken to minimize the risks and that all other conditions for the ethical conduct of research are met. There may also be cases in which, although the knowledge to be gained is of great importance, an IRB judges that the risks to participants are too great to allow the study to be conducted. For a study to make a significant contribution to medical knowledge, it must be a well-designed, scientifically rigorous study with an appropriate sample size. Thus, in reviewing research protocols, IRBs must assess the extent to which studies are designed in such a way that they have the potential to yield generalizable knowledge. It is not permissible to expose participants to risks and burdens if the study is likely to be of no benefit. While IRBs are not strictly scientific review committees, scientific rigor and the potential scientific value of studies are pertinent to determining whether proposed research is ethical.

A second criterion for IRB review and approval concerns the selection of research participants. The benefits and burdens of participating in research should not be disproportionately borne by particular groups or classes. Research on conditions that affect only particular groups may require exclusion of other participants, but for conditions that affect a wide range of persons, participants should not be selected in a way that is likely to result in unbalanced participant pools. The goal is not equal or statistically proportionate representation in research. The obligation to ensure that participant selection is just and fair is more nuanced. The goal is to ensure that no class of persons, such as the poor or minorities, is being recruited because they typically are more willing participants, for example. This requirement is explicitly outlined in *The Belmont Report*:

> Against this historical background [of abuses in biomedical research], it can be seen how conceptions of justice are relevant to research involving human subjects. For example, the selection of research subjects needs to be scrutinized in order to determine whether some classes (e.g., welfare patients, particular racial and ethnic minorities, or persons confined to institutions) are being systematically selected simply because of their easy availability, their compromised position, or their manipulability, rather than for reasons directly related to the problem being studied.
>
> (1979: B.3)

Third, studies must include appropriate plans to obtain informed consent from research participants (or their legal surrogates) (see 45CFR46.116) and to document their informed consent (see 45CFR46.117). There are circumstances under which studies may proceed without traditional documentation of informed consent, and some may even proceed without obtaining informed consent at all. Those exceptions will be noted later. Generally, however, participants (or their surrogates) must freely and voluntarily give their informed consent to enroll in a study and the consent must be documented. To ensure that their consent is free and voluntary, investigators must establish a mechanism for obtaining informed consent that does not restrict potential participants' ability to consider the study and to ask questions. Actions, statements, or circumstances that, even if not intended to be coercive or unduly influential, may be perceived by certain subjects as such must be avoided. Many have argued that providing payments to subjects that are high enough to make persons feel as if they could not reasonably refuse to participate can be coercive or unduly influential. Thus, IRBs must assess whether the compensation investigators intend to offer subjects is commensurate with the level of burden, such as time, discomfort, and cost, which subjects are asked to bear. IRBs may ask investigators to justify the level of compensation being offered to ensure that it is appropriate.[15]

In order to be sufficiently informed to consent, potential participants must understand that they are being asked to participate in research, what kind of study they are being asked to enroll in, and the purpose of the study, what will be required of them if they choose to participate, the risks and benefits associated with the study, the discomforts they may expect as participants, and what alternatives exist to participating in the study. In addition, persons should be told what treatment and compensation, if any, is available should they be injured as a result of their participation. They should be given the names and telephone numbers of persons to contact if they have questions regarding the study itself or their rights. Finally, it should be made clear to persons that by enrolling in a study they are not committed to remaining in the study and they may terminate their participation at any time. The CFR identifies additional elements that may need to be disclosed in the informed consent process depending on the nature of the research, including the number of subjects to participate in the study, the possibility that there are unforeseeable risks associated with the study, and the costs that the participants may incur as a result of enrolling in the study.

When the research subject is a child under the age of 18, one or both parents or a legal guardian must give informed consent. Depending on their age, children may be asked to assent to participate in the study. Research protocols involving children must be categorized by IRBs into 1 of 4 categories; the permissibility of conducting the research and the consent requirements vary by category.

The importance of informed consent cannot be underestimated, particularly in light of the history of abuses in biomedical research. The extent to which persons can adequately understand the proposed study and the risks it imposes is always of concern, for there is evidence that individuals often have poor risk-assessment and risk-analysis skills. A number of studies have shown that many people lack a basic understanding of statistics and probabilities which are essential to assessing risk (Kovera *et al.* 1999; Lehman and Nisbett 1990; Nisbett and Ross 1980; Tversky and Kahneman 1981; Yamagishi 1997). Moreover, individuals interpret the same information regarding risk differently, and their understanding of risk varies based on how the information is presented (Edwards *et al.* 1998, 2001, 2002; Gurm and Litaker 2000; O'Connor 1989). A further problem involves the extent to which persons understand (or misunderstand) the benefits of participating in research. In designing consent materials, investigators must pay special attention to minimizing the possibility that potential participants will misunderstand the purpose of bio-medical research and see it as a mere extension of their routine therapeutic clinical care or as a way to obtain better care. This is a problem that the IRBs must consider in reviewing consent documents. Considerable attention has been given to this prob-lem in the bioethics literature. For example, Appelbaum and his colleagues identi-fied the problem of "therapeutic misconception" among some research participants enrolled in psychiatric studies (1982, 1987). It has been documented in other sub-ject populations, such as persons enrolled in Phase I oncology trials (Daugherty *et al.* 2000; Yoder *et al.* 1997). Therapeutic misconception refers to research participants' failure to see the distinction between research and the clinical/therapeutic setting. A related but distinct set of issues was identified by Sam Horng and Christine Grady (2003). They distinguished Appelbaum's therapeutic misconception from therapeu-tic misestimation and therapeutic optimism. Therapeutic misestimation refers to participants' overestimation of the benefits of research participation and/or under-estimation of the risks of participation. They concluded that it was sometimes but not always ethically problematic. Finally, therapeutic optimism refers to participants' hope that research participation will benefit them. This optimism, Horng and Grady argue, is not ethically problematic.

Despite the importance of obtaining informed consent for most biomedical research, there are recognized exceptions that allow IRBs to approve altered consent procedures or to waive the informed consent requirement altogether. Specifically, waivers of consent may be granted when an IRB finds and documents that:

(1) the research or demonstration project is to be conducted by or subject to the approval of state or local government officials and is designed to study, evaluate, or otherwise examine: (i) public benefit or service programs; (ii) pro-cedures for obtaining benefits or services under those programs; (iii) possible changes in or alternatives to those programs or procedures; or (iv) possible changes in methods or levels of payment for benefits or services under those programs; and
(2) the research could not practicably be carried out without the waiver or alteration of consent procedures.

(45CFR46.116c)

Or, an IRB finds and documents that:

(1) the research involves no more than minimal risk to the subjects;
(2) the waiver or alteration will not adversely affect the rights and welfare of the subjects;
(3) the research could not practicably be carried out without the waiver or alteration; and
(4) whenever appropriate, the subjects will be provided with additional pertinent information after participation.

(45CFR46.116d)

Chart reviews, for example, typically qualify for waivers of informed consent, although sometimes physicians whose charts are to be reviewed are informed of the intent to review their charts and are given an opportunity to disallow use of their charts. Research that involves analysis of previously obtained tissue samples, especially de-identified samples, also is usually conducted with a waiver of consent.

In addition to ensuring that the investigators have an appropriate plan to obtain informed consent, IRBs must also ensure that their plans for documenting the consent are appropriate. Most research requires that participants (or their legal representatives) sign a written consent form. In most cases, this form contains all the elements that are to be provided as part of obtaining consent as noted earlier, including the nature and purpose of the research, the benefits and burdens of participation, the costs to participants, alternatives to participation, and so on. The consent form is not intended to replace oral communication with potential subjects, and the expectation is that subjects will be provided the information orally in a setting in which they may ask questions. The consent form is intended to document the process, and a copy of the form is to be provided to subjects for future reference. Despite the circumstance that the written consent document is intended to supplement the information provided to subjects and not be the focal point of the informed consent process, it is the element of the informed consent process to which most IRBs give the greatest attention. Consent documents are to be written in simple lay language that a wide range of subjects can be expected to understand. Technical terms should be avoided and, where used, should be explained in simple language. Although the OHRP prefers that all the information pertinent to a study be made available to subjects in a consent document whenever possible (OHRP 2001: chapter 3), the CFR provides for the possibility of what is known as a "short form" consent document (45CFR46.117b2). In some institutions this option is exercised when prospective subjects do not read English and it is not possible to translate the entire consent document into a language they can read. Short forms include a statement saying that all of the information necessary for persons to give their free and informed consent has been provided orally to the participant or the participant's legal representative. This form is then signed by the subject. Investigators also must present to the IRB for review and approval a summary of the information they plan to provide orally to prospective participants. The oral presentation must be witnessed by a third party who is then asked to sign both the short form and the summary, attesting to the fact that all the information was in fact given to the subject. The person who obtains the participant's consent must also sign the summary. A copy of both the short form itself and the summary must be given to the participant.

Despite the importance generally given to the documentation of informed consent, there are cases in which consent is obtained only orally and persons are not asked to sign a document, though they may be given a summary page with information regarding the study. Waivers for obtaining signed consent may be issued when an IRB finds and documents that one of two circumstances pertains. First are cases in which a signed form would be the only link that existed between a participant and a study and where the principal risk of participating in the study is a harm that would come from a loss of confidentiality. In those cases, subjects are asked whether or not they wish to sign a consent form and those who choose not to document their consent are not obligated to do so. One example of a study that might be approved with a waiver of consent under this provision is a study in which human immunodeficiency virus (HIV) positive persons are interviewed about their experience of living with HIV. The greatest risk of participating in the study may be a loss of confidentiality, and if their names are recorded nowhere but on a signed consent form, the only opportunity for their name to be made known is through the signed form. The second reason for waiving the requirement that informed consent be documented with a signed form is if the research is of no more than minimal risk and the research involves no procedures that would otherwise require a written consent (45CFR46.117c).

A fourth principal requirement for the ethical conduct of research is that, when appropriate, investigators design and implement data safety monitoring plans (45CFR46.111). There may be risks associated with the use of a drug or a device that are not known prior to a study. As a study progresses, however, such risks may be identified with proper monitoring of adverse events. In some cases, new risks may require that all currently enrolled participants be told of the risk so that they can decide whether to continue their participation. They may be asked to sign an amendment to the original consent form acknowledging that they have been informed of and understand the new risks. The consent process for new participants should include information regarding the newly identified risks. In other cases, the risks may be serious enough to warrant termination of the trial. Another reason for premature termination of a trial may be clear evidence that certain participants are doing significantly better or much worse than others. Without appropriate and effective implementation of plans to monitor data throughout a trial, this information is not available. The monitoring of clinical trials is discussed further in Chapter 5 on randomized controlled trials.

Sometimes it is not until after a trial has ended that investigators learn that taking a particular drug or using a given device increases individuals' risk for developing other problems. For example, what initially appeared to be a gene therapy breakthrough in the treatment of severe combined immunodeficiency syndrome (SCID) was linked with leukemia in research participants thirty months after the trial (Hacein-Bey-Abina *et al.* 2003). In the same way that it is important to report newly identified risks to currently enrolled participants, it is important to inform participants of a trial that has ended if they are at increased risk as a result of having participated in a study. This is not written into the CFR but has been the subject of discussion (Fernandez *et al.* 2003). Post-study data safety monitoring plans that call for informing former participants of risks may become the standard of practice in biomedical research.

Fifth, when conducting studies in which information that could be linked to participants is collected or used, investigators must take appropriate measures to protect the privacy and confidentiality of those persons. When the Health Insurance Portability and Accountability Act (HIPAA) took effect on April 14, 2003, investigators became responsible for a new level of privacy protection. Ensuring that studies conform to HIPAA regulations has become a new element in the IRB review process at many institutions.[16]

Finally, when studies include populations considered vulnerable by the federal government, such as children, pregnant women, fetuses, neonates, prisoners, the mentally disabled, the educationally disadvantaged, and the economically disadvantaged, the DHHS requires that additional measures be taken to protect their rights and their welfare. Although some of this is left to the judgment and interpretation of investigators and IRBs, there are specific regulations governing the participation of children, prisoners, pregnant women, fetuses, and neonates in research.

Subpart B of 45CFR46 addresses the participation of pregnant women, fetuses, and neonates in biomedical research. A number of important additional elements must be included to allow for the participation of pregnant women in research, but the most important elements concern consent and the termination of a pregnancy. When the research has the prospect of directly benefiting only the pregnant woman, or both the pregnant woman and the fetus, or neither the pregnant woman nor the fetus, but it poses no greater than minimal risk to the fetus, the pregnant woman may consent to participate. However, studies in which only the fetus may benefit require that both the pregnant woman and the father give their consent (unless the father is unavailable, incompetent, or temporarily incapacitated, or the pregnancy is the result of rape or incest) (45CFR46.204). In addition, federal regulations make it impermissible for investigators to offer any type of inducement to a woman to terminate a pregnancy, to be involved in any decision to terminate a pregnancy, and to make judgments regarding the viability of a neonate.

When prisoners are to be part of a study, the regulations require a number of additional safeguards. Some of the most important regulations concern the composition of the IRB reviewing a study, the risks, and benefits of studies, subject selection procedures, and the reasons for using prisoners in the proposed study. The majority of IRB members must not be affiliated with the prison(s) to be involved in the research and there must be at least one prisoner or prisoner representative on the IRB. A prisoner representative is someone who has worked with the prison population sufficiently so that he or she may represent the interests of prisoners. Extra care must be taken to ensure that participation in research would not give prisoners access to any opportunities, benefits, or experiences that would be a significant improvement over life in prison without study participation. This is to avoid unduly influencing them to participate or to discount the risks of participation. The risks must not be greater than those to which the IRB would be willing to expose non-prisoners. Participants must be selected in a way that is fair to all prisoners who meet the inclusion criteria and prison officials should not be permitted to arbitrarily influence the selection process (45CFR46.305). Finally, only when the research proposed is in one of the following areas may the study use prisoners as subjects:

(A) study of the possible causes, effects, and processes of incarceration, and of criminal behavior...
(B) study of prisons as institutional structures or of prisoners as incarcerated persons...
(C) research on conditions particularly affecting prisoners as a class (e.g., vaccine trials and other research on hepatitis which is much more prevalent in

prisons than elsewhere; and research on social and psychological problems such as alcoholism, drug addiction, and sexual assaults) provided that... the Secretary [of the Department of Health and Human Services approves of the study] ...

(D) research on practices, both innovative and accepted, which have the intent and reasonable probability of improving the health or well-being of the subject. In cases in which those studies require the assignment of prisoners in a manner consistent with protocols approved by the IRB to control groups which may not benefit from the research, the study may proceed only after the Secretary [approves the study].

(45CFR46.306a2)

The final portion of the DHHS regulations governing research on human subjects, Subpart D, pertains to children. In addition to the regulations that govern all research on human persons, research on children must meet more stringent restrictions. There are four categories of research involving children. First, when the proposed research poses no more than minimal risk to children, a parent or legal guardian must consent to the child's participation and, children who are mature enough to understand what they are being asked to do must give their assent (45CFR46.404). The age at which children are asked to give their assent varies, but many believe that children as young as 6 or 7 may give assent and most recognize that by the age of 10 children should be asked to give assent to their participation.[17] Some IRBs ask investigators to obtain assent from those children who appear mature enough to provide it rather than requiring assent of all children above a certain age. Second, when research poses greater than minimal risk to children but presents them with the prospect of direct benefit, children may participate provided that the expected benefits outweigh the risks, that the risk–benefit ratio is at least as good as that of the alternatives to participating in research (e.g., non-research therapies already available), at least one parent or legal guardian gives consent, and, when appropriate, the assent of the child is sought and obtained (45CFR46.405). A third category of research involving children is that which poses greater than minimal risk and no prospect of direct benefit to the participants but is "likely to yield generalizable knowledge about the subjects' disorder or condition which is of vital importance for the understanding or amelioration of the subjects' disorder or condition" (45CFR46.406). Such research is permissible only when the risk is only slightly greater than minimal and "the intervention or procedure presents experiences to subjects that are reasonably commensurate with those inherent in their actual or expected medical, dental, psychological, social, or educational situations" (45CFR46.406). Such research requires the consent of both parents and, when appropriate, the child's assent. The consent of only one parent is required if the other parent is "deceased, unknown, incompetent, or not reasonably available, or when only one parent has legal responsibility for the care and custody of the child" (45CFR46.408).[18] The fourth category of research on children is research that poses greater than minimal risk, no prospect of direct benefit, and is not likely to yield generalizable knowledge about a child's condition. To be approved, such research must be reviewed by the Secretary of DHHS. If, after consulting with experts, the Secretary determines that in addition to meeting all the requirements of sound, ethical research, the research "presents a reasonable opportunity to further the understanding, prevention, or alleviation of a serious problem affecting the health or welfare of children" (45CFR46.407), then the research may be permitted. As with category three research, both parents must give their consent, unless certain conditions are met, and, when appropriate, children should give their assent. Children who are wards of the state may participate in research only if the research is "related to their status as wards or is conducted in schools, camps, hospitals institutions, or similar settings in which the majority of children involved as subjects are not wards" (45CFR46.409).

Interest in including children in research has increased in recent years as pharmaceutical companies seek to label their products for pediatric use. In 2001, the US Congress passed the Best Pharmaceuticals for Children Act, providing additional avenues to request and fund research on pharmaceutical products in children. It was signed into law by President Bush in January 2002 (PL 107–09). In December 2003, Congress passed the Pediatric Research Equity Act (PL 108–55) giving the FDA the authority to require that drugs be studied in children. The principal scientific reason for encouraging such research is that many pharmaceutical products have not been tested in children but are routinely used in pediatric populations. Studies to determine appropriate pediatric dosing, to establish drug safety, and to identify side effects or other problems that a product might cause in children can increase medical safety for children.

Emphasis on the role of IRBs should not be taken to mean that only IRBs are responsible for ensuring that research is conducted in responsible and ethical manner. That burden falls on all who are involved in the process, including investigators, co-investigators, research assistants, and research coordinators. It is the responsibility of IRBs to ensure that individuals responsible for conducting research on human persons do so in an ethical and responsible fashion. IRBs work toward this end by reviewing studies before they begin and by reviewing their progress at least once per year. In addition, IRBs may request audits of studies to assess the extent to which they are being conducted in an ethical and responsible manner.

As with all areas of health-care ethics, research ethics is more than merely complying with legal and regulatory requirements. Often laws, policies, and regulations require careful interpretation, judgment, and application by investigators and members of IRBs.

This chapter introduced the widely accepted standards that must be met to conduct ethical research on human subjects as these standards have been enumerated in documents concerning research ethics, particularly the CFR in the United States. The remainder of this volume addresses important contemporary issues in research ethics, ranging from particular types of trials and areas of research, research on specific (vulnerable) groups, institutional management of conflicts of interest in research, and the presentation and use of data.

Recent concerns over bioterrorism have led to renewed interest in testing smallpox vaccines. This, along with ongoing efforts to develop a vaccine against HIV, have brought to the forefront the ethics of vaccine research, a topic addressed by Christine Grady in Chapter 2. Lisa Parker and Lauren Matukaitis Broyles consider a wide range of issues raised by various types of genetics research, including mapping studies and gene transfer trials in Chapter 3. Ana Smith Iltis' Chapter 5 on randomized controlled trials addresses the permissibility of initiating, conducting, monitoring, and stopping randomized controlled trials in general and attends to the special concerns raised by randomized, placebo-controlled trials. Gerard Magill, in Chapter 4 on stem cell research, situates the contemporary controversy within a broader study of the social and political factors and issues that frame the "stem cell wars" today. Included in his chapter is a discussion of ethical concerns related to stem cell research, such as fetal tissue research and human cloning.

While most of the volume focuses on biomedical research on human persons, behavioral and social sciences (BSS) research is subject to the same federal regulations that govern biomedical research. James DuBois provides an insightful analysis of the principal areas of ethical concern in conducting an overseeing BSS research.

Other chapters in the volume focus on research conducted on particular categories of persons widely recognized as vulnerable. Loretta Kopelman's contribution on research involving infants, children, and adolescents discusses, among other things, the implications of *The Belmont Report*'s principles for the ethical conduct of pediatric research. In Chapter 8 on research in the developing world, David Resnik discusses the highly controversial placebo-controlled studies conducted in developing nations during the 1990s to test the efficacy of a regimen for reducing the transmission of HIV from pregnant women to their children that would cost less than the standard of care in the United States. His analysis points to many of the ethical issues posed by research in the developing world.

Chapter 9 on conflicts of interest by Mark J. Cherry addresses a concern that has taken a prominent position in recent years. Investigators conducting research can have two main kinds of conflicts of interest: financial ones and nonfinancial ones (e.g., role conflicts between their status as clinicians and researchers). Much attention has been given recently to financial conflicts of interest, and Cherry's chapter offers a landscape of the current controversies and concerns. Finally, Griffin Trotter in Chapter 10 considers a set of issues not often discussed as a matter of research ethics, but nonetheless important and serious: the role of investigators, non-investigator physician "experts," and the media in choosing which studies should be presented to the public and when, in interpreting data for public consumption, and in announcing the implications of such data for clinical care. These parties have significant influence on what the public hears and on how the public understands study results. Failure to interpret studies responsibly, to present both positive and negative results and to situate benefits alongside the risks of new interventions, can lead to skewed expectations and, sometimes, to demands for harmful or inappropriate interventions.

Notes

1 According to the CFR, research is "a systematic investigation, including research development, testing, and evaluation, designed to develop or contribute to generalizable

knowledge" (45CFR46.102). Research can involve retrospective (e.g., chart review) and prospective (e.g., clinical trial) assessment of interventions.

2 It should be noted that there are serious abuses in the history of research involving human persons that are not discussed at length here and that typically are not cited as pivotal events in the development of research ethics. The failure to discuss these cases in further detail here should not be taken as an indication that these abuses were not serious. Rather, they are not discussed here because they did not play a major role in the emergence of the federal government's interest in regulating research. I cannot speculate on the reasons for this here. But it is worth noting that abuses beyond those often cited existed, and such abuses should not continue to be ignored in the literature. One example of such research is the medical and surgical experimentation carried out on slave women in the United States, which led to major developments in gynecology. For an insightful discussion and analysis of this research, see Nelson (2005).

3 Readers should note that individual states may further regulate research.

4 The details of these and other experiments have been recounted in the literature. No description I could attempt here would be adequate. For a discussion of the experiments and for an analysis of the implications of those experiments for bioethics, see *When Medicine Went Mad: Bioethics and the Holocaust* (Caplan 1992). See also the report by Leo Alexander, a US Army Medical Corps major, who was assigned to analyze some of the records found on the experiments (Alexander 1946) and the transcripts of the Nuremberg Trials (*Trials of War Criminals before the Nuremberg Military Tribunals under Control Council Law*, October 1946–April 1949. Washington, DC: US GPO, 1949–1953).

5 One of the issues that emerged after the Nuremberg Trials that is not addressed by the Nuremberg Code concerns the permissibility of using the data generated in the Nazi experiments. Much of the debate has turned on two questions. First, are the data scientifically valid? If they are not, then the value of the data is diminished sufficiently that interest in using it should be eliminated. However, if there are data that are valid and that might be useful, a second question emerges: is it ethically permissible to use the data? Both questions have been thoroughly debated in both the scientific and the bioethics literature. For further discussion of the scientific and ethical debate on this issue, see Caplan (1992), especially the chapters by Pozos, Berger, Pozos and Katz, Freedman, and Greene. See also Berger (1994), Bleich (1991), Cohen (1990), Folker and Hafner (1989), Gaylin (1989), Martin (1986), Moe (1984), Mostow (1993–1994), Post (1991), Rosenbaum (1989), Rosner *et al.* (1991), Schafer (1986), Seidelman (1988), Sheldon and Whitely (1989).

6 See Katz (1972: 9–65) for further discussion of the Jewish Chronic Disease Hospital study.

7 Like the United States, many other countries have a history of abuses in biomedical research and have developed their own standards for the ethical conduct of biomedical research. For example, during the 1960s and 1970s in New Zealand, women with in situ cervical cancer were left untreated to follow the progression of the disease (Brody 1998: 33). Many of the women developed invasive cancers and died. The fact that a number of the women had not given consent to be research subjects, that it was already well known that untreated in situ cervical cancer would progress and lead to death, and that the study was not scientifically well designed and had not been subjected to adequate scientific and ethical review led a judge to recommend improvements in the oversight of human subjects research in New Zealand. The recommendations were adopted by New Zealand's Department of Health and have continued to shape the conduct of ethics committees there (McNeil 1993: 76–78).

8 See Jonsen (1998: 99–106) for a historical account of the Commission's activities and its members.

9 The history of research scandals presented above suggests that participation in research as a subject carries significant risks and that these risks often have been borne by what might be classified as vulnerable populations, including imprisoned persons, institutionalized children, and the poor. However, in recent years, there has been a surge in interest in participating in research, particularly in research for certain diseases or conditions. Among some there is a sense that patients have a right to participate in research, especially

when they suffer from a condition for which no effective treatment exists. For a discussion of this changing perspective on biomedical research, see *When Science Offers Salvation* by Rebecca Dresser (2001).

10 See 56 Federal Register 28002–28032, June 18, 1991. For a comparison of the CFR and FDA regulations, see *OHRP Guidebook*, 2001, chapter 2. The departments that share the Common Rule are: Department of Agriculture, Department of Energy, National Aeronautics and Space Administration, Department of Commerce, Consumer Product Safety Commission, Agency for International Development, Department of Housing and Urban Development, Department of Justice, Department of Defense, Department of Education, Department of Veterans Affairs, Environmental Protection Agency, Department of Health and Human Services, National Science Foundation, Department of Transportation, the Social Security Administration, and the Central Intelligence Agency. The DHHS regulations appear at 45CFR46 and are the most often cited reference to the Common Rule. The other agencies have identical regulations that appear elsewhere in the CFR. The DHHS has additional regulations governing research on prisoners, pregnant women, fetuses, neonates, and children that appear in subparts of 45CFR46. The FDA regulations appear at 21CFR50 and 21CFR56.

11 See 45CFR46.101 and 102e and 21CFR50.1 for further details concerning research that is subject to the CFR. A federal-wide assurance is a contract between institutions and the federal government in which institutions commit themselves to protecting human subjects by ensuring that all studies conform to the federal regulations governing human subjects research.

12 The circumstance that there is some human subjects research conducted in the United States that is not subject to federal regulations has been the subject of controversy. Some have argued that all research should be subject to the conditions set forth in the regulations (see, e.g., National Bioethics Advisory Commission 2001).

13 For further discussion of these issues, see Boyce (2001), Cohen (2001), Green *et al.* (2002), Knox (2001), McGee (2001), Stolberg (2001), and White (1999).

14 The nine categories are printed in the *Federal Register* (63FR60364–60367, November 9, 1998) and are available online at: http://www.hhs.gov/ohrp/humansubjects/guidance/expedited98.htm (last accessed July 17, 2005).

15 For further discussion of payments to subjects, see Casarett *et al.* (2002), Dickert and Grady (1999), Grady (2001), Lemmens and Miller (2003), McNeill (1997), Schonfeld *et al.* (2003), Tishler and Bartholomae (2002), and Wilkinson and Moore (1997).

16 For further discussion of privacy regulations and the conduct of research, see Amatayakul (2003), Annas (2002), Kamoi and Hodge (2004), and Kulynych and Korn (2002).

17 For further discussion of assent in pediatric research, see Bartholome (1995), Brody *et al.* (2003), Nelson and Reynolds (2003), Ondrusek *et al.* (1998), Rossi *et al.* (2003), Sterling and Walco (2003), and Tait *et al.* (2003).

18 Some have expressed concern that this category of research permits children with a disorder or condition to be exposed to more risk than healthy children even when a study poses no prospect of direct benefit. For further discussion, see Ross (2003).

Bibliography

Advisory Committee on Human Radiation Experiments (ACHRE), Department of Energy (1995) *Advisory Committee on Human Radiation Experiments Final Report*, Washington, DC: Government Printing Office.

Alexander, L. (1946) *The Treatment of Shock from Prolonged Exposure to Cold Especially in Water. Item #24, #350*, Washington, DC: Office of Publication Board, Department of Commerce.

Amatayakul, M. (2003) "Another Layer of Regulations: Research under HIPAA," *Journal of American Health Information Management Association*, 74(1): 16A–D.

Amundsen, D. (1981a) "Casuistry and Professional Obligations: The Regulation of Physicians by the Court of Conscience in the Late Middle Ages, Part I," *Transactions and Studies of the College of Physicians of Philadelphia*, 3(2): 22–29.

——(1981b) "Casuistry and Professional Obligations: The Regulation of Physicians by the Court of Conscience in the Late Middle Ages, Part II," *Transactions and Studies of the College of Physicians of Philadelphia*, 3(3): 93–112.

Annas, G.J. (2002) "Medical Privacy and Medical Research—Judging the New Federal Regulations," *New England Journal of Medicine*, 346(3): 216–20.

Appelbaum, P.S., Roth, L.H., Lidz, C.W., Benson, P., and Winslade, W. (1987) "False Hopes and Best Data: Consent to Research and the Therapeutic Misconception," *Hastings Center Report*, 12(2): 20–24.

Appelbaum, P.S., Roth, L.H., and Lidz, C.W. (1982) "The Therapeutic Misconception: Informed Consent in Psychiatric Research," *International Journal of Law and Psychiatry*, 5: 319–29.

Bartholome, W.G. (1995) "Informed Consent, Parental Permission, and Assent in Pediatric Practice," *Pediatrics*, 96(5 Pt 1): 981–82.

Beecher, H.K. (1966) "Ethics and Clinical Research," *New England Journal of Medicine*, 274: 1354–60.

Berger, R.L. (1994) "Ethics in Scientific Communication: Study of a Problem Case," *Journal of Medical Ethics*, 20(4): 207–11.

——(1992) "Nazi Science: Comments on the Validation of the Dachau Human Hypothermia Experiments," in A. Caplan (ed.) *When Medicine Went Mad: Bioethics and the Holocaust* (pp. 109–33), Totowa, NJ: Humana Press.

Bleich, J.D. (1991) "Utilization of Scientific Data Obtained through Immoral Experimentation: Survey of Recent Halakhic Literature," *Tradition*, 26: 65–79.

Boyce, N. (2001) "And Now, Ethics for Sale?: Bioethicists and Big Bucks. Problem City?," *US News and World Report*, July 30, 18–19.

Brody, B.A. (1998) *The Ethics of Biomedical Research: An International Perspective*, New York: Oxford University Press.

Brody, J.L., Scherer, D.G., Annett, R.D., and Pearson-Bish, M. (2003) "Voluntary Assent in Biomedical Research with Adolescents: A Comparison of Parent and Adolescent Views," *Ethics & Behavior*, 13(1): 79–95.

Caplan, A. (ed.) (1992) *When Medicine Went Mad: Bioethics and the Holocaust*, Totowa, NJ: Humana Press.

Casarett, D., Karlawish, J., and Asch, D.A. (2002) "Paying Hypertension Research Subjects: Fair Compensation or Undue Inducement?," *Journal of General Internal Medicine*, 17: 650–52.

Cherry, M.C. (2002) "Medical Fact and Ulcer Disease: A Study in Scientific Controversy Resolution," *History and Philosophy of the Life Sciences*, 24: 249–73.

Code of Federal Regulations (CFR), Online available: http://www.gpoaccess.gov/cfr/index.html (accessed September 7, 2004).

Cohen, B. (1990) "The Ethics of Using Medical Data from Nazi Experiments," *Journal of Halacha and Contemporary Society*, 19: 103–26.

Cohen, C. (2001) "Letter to the Editor: Ethical Issues in Embryonic Stem Cell Research," *Journal of the American Medical Association*, 285: 1439.

Cohen, P. (1998) "The Placebo is not Dead: Three Historical Vignettes," *IRB: A Review of Human Subjects Research*, 20(2–3): 6–8.

Council for International Organizations of Medical Sciences (CIOMS) (1993/2002) *International Ethical Guidelines for Biomedical Research Involving Human Subjects*, Geneva: CIOMS.

—— (1982) *Human Experimentation and Medical Ethics*, Geneva: CIOMS.

Daugherty, C.K., Danik, D.M., Janish, L., and Ratain, M.J. (2000) "Quantitative Analysis of Ethical Issues in Phase I Trials: A Survey Interview Study of 144 Advanced Cancer Patients," *IRB: A Review of Human Subjects Research*, 22(3): 6–14.

Dickert, N. and Grady, C. (1999) "What's the Price of a Research Subject? Approaches to Payment for Research Participation," *The New England Journal of Medicine*, 341: 198–203.

Dresser, R. (2001) *When Science Offers Salvation*, New York: Oxford University Press.

Edwards, A., Elwyn, G., and Mulley, A. (2002) "Explaining Risks: Turning Numerical Data into Meaningful Pictures," *British Medical Journal*, 324: 827–30.

Edwards, A., Elwyn, G., Matthews, E., and Pill, R. (2001) "Presenting Risk Information— A Review of the Effects of 'Framing' and Other Manipulations on Patient Outcomes," *Journal of Health Communication*, 6: 61–82.

Edwards, A., Matthews, E., Pill, R., and Bloor, M. (1998) "Communication about Risk: The Responses of Primary Care Professionals to Standardizing the 'Language of Risk' and Communication Tools," *Family Practice*, 15(4): 301–07.

"Federal Policy for the Protection of Human Subjects; Notices and Rules" (1991) 56 *Federal Register* 28002–28032 (June 18).

Fernandez, C.V., Kodish, E., and Weijer, C. (2003) "Informing Study Participants of Research Results: An Ethical Imperative," *IRB: A Review of Human Subjects Research*, 25(3): 12–19.

Folker, B. and Hafner, A.W. (1989) "Nazi Data: Dissociation from Evil," Commentary, *Hastings Center Report*, 19(4): 17–18.

Freedman, B. (1992) "Moral Analysis and the Use of Nazi Experimental Results," in A. Caplan (ed.) *When Medicine Went Mad: Bioethics and the Holocaust* (pp. 141–54), Totowa, NJ: Humana Press.

Gaylin, W. (1989) "Nazi Data: Dissociation from Evil," Commentary, *Hastings Center Report*, 19(4): 18.

Grady, C. (2001) "Money for Research Participation: Does it Jeopardize Informed Consent?," *American Journal of Bioethics*, 1(2): 40–44.

Green, R.M., DeVries, K.O., Bernstein, J., Goodman, K.W., Kaufmann, R., Kiessling, A.A., Levin, S.R., Moss, S.L., and Tauer, C.A. (2002) "Overseeing Research on Therapeutic Cloning: A Private Ethics Board Responds to its Critics," *Hastings Center Report*, 32(3): 27–33.

Greene, V.W. (1992) "Can Scientists Use Information Derived from the Concentration Camps? Ancient Answers to New Questions," in A. Caplan (ed.) *When Medicine Went Mad: Bioethics and the Holocaust* (pp. 155–74), Totowa, NJ: Humana Press.

Gurm, H.S. and Litaker, D.G. (2000) "Framing Procedural Risks to Patients: Is 99% Safe the Same as a Risk of 1 in 100?," *Academic Medicine*, 75: 840–42.

Hacein-Bey-Abina, S., von Kalle, C., Schmidt, M., Le Deist, F., Wulffraat, N., McIntyre, E., Radford, I., Villeval, J.-L., Fraser, C., Cavazzana-Calvo, M., and Fischer, A. (2003) "A Serious Adverse Event after Successful Gene Therapy for X-linked Severe Combined Immunodeficiency," *New England Journal of Medicine*, 348(3): 255–56.

Health Insurance Portability and Accountability Act of 1996. PL 104–91.

Horng, S. and Grady, C. (2003) "Misunderstanding in Clinical Research: Distinguishing Therapeutic Misconception, Therapeutic Misestimation, and Therapeutic Optimism," *IRB: Ethics and Human Research*, 25: 11–16.

Jones, J.H. (1981) *Bad Blood: The Tuskegee Syphilis Experiment*, New York: The Free Press.

Jonsen, A. (1998) *The Birth of Bioethics*, New York: Oxford University Press.

Kamoie, B. and Hodge, Jr, J.G. (2004) "HIPPAA's Implications for Public Health Policy and Practice: Guidance from the CDC," *Public Health Reports*, 119(2): 216–19.

Katz, J. (1972) *Experimentation with Human Beings*, New York: Russell Sage Foundation.

Knox, A. (2001) "Ethicist Spurs Debate on Biological Research," *Philadelphia Inquirer*, July 17.

Kovera, M.B., McAuliff, B.D., and Hebert, K.S. (1999) "Reasoning about Scientific Evidence: The Effects of Juror Gender and Evidence Quality on Juror Decisions in a Hostile Work Environment Case," *Journal of Applied Psychology*, 84: 362–75.

Kulynych, J. and Korn, D. (2002) "The Effect of the New Federal Medical–Privacy Rule on Research," *New England Journal of Medicine*, 346(3): 201–04.

Lehman, D.R. and Nisbett, R.E. (1990) "A Longitudinal Study of the Effects of Undergraduate Training on Reasoning," *Developmental Psychology*, 26: 952–60.

Lemmens, T. and Miller, P.B. (2003) "The Human Subjects Trade: Ethical and Legal Issues Surrounding Recruitment Incentives," *Journal of Law, Medicine & Ethics*, 31: 398–418.

McGee, G. (2001) "Testimony before the U.S. Senate Committee on Appropriations," August 1. Online available: http://appropriations.senate.gov/releases/record.cfm?id=178311 (accessed July 2, 2004).

McNeill, P. (1997) "Paying People to Participate in Research: Why Not?," *Bioethics*, 11(5): 390–96.

——(1993) *The Ethics and Politics of Human Experimentation*, Cambridge: Cambridge University Press.

Martin, R.M. (1986) "Using Nazi Scientific Data," *Dialogue*, 25: 403–11.

Moe, K. (1984) "Should the Nazi Research Data be Cited?," *Hastings Center Report*, 14(6): 5–7.

Mostow, P. (1993–1994) "Like Building on Top of Auschwitz: On the Symbolic Meaning of Using Data from the Nazi Experiments, and on Nonuse as a Form of Memorial," *Journal of Law and Religion*, 10(2): 403–31.

National Bioethics Advisory Commission (2001) *Ethical and Policy Issues in Research Involving Human Participants*, Rockville, MD: NBAC. Online available: www.georgetown.edu/research/nrcbl/nbac/pubs/oversight.pdf (accessed September 25, 2004).

National Commission for the Protection of Human Subjects of Biomedical and Behavioral Research (1979) *The Belmont Report*, Washington, DC: Government Printing Office.

Nelson, C. (2005) "American Husbandry: Legal Norms Impacting the Production of Reproduction," *Colombia Journal of Gender and Law*, 15(1).

Nelson, R.M. and Reynolds, W.W. (2003) "Child Assent and Parental Permission: A Comment on Tait's 'Do They Understand?'," *Anesthesiology*, 98(3): 597–98.

Nisbett, R. and Ross, L. (1980) *Human Inference: Strategies and Shortcomings of Social Judgment*, Englewood Cliffs, NJ: Prentice Hall.

Nuremberg Code (1947/1949) *The Nuremberg Code: Trials of War Criminals before the Nuremberg Military Tribunals under Control Council Law 2(10)*, Washington, DC: US Government Printing Office.

O'Connor, A.M. (1989) "Effect of Framing and Level of Probability on Patients' Preferences for Cancer Chemotherapy," *Journal of Clinical Epidemiology*, 42: 119–26.

Office of Human Research Protections (OHRP) (2001) *IRB Guidebook*, Washington, DC: Government Printing Office. Online available: http://www.med.umich.edu/irbmed/OPRR-IRBguidebook/contents.htm (accessed July 29, 2004).

Ondrusek, N., Abramovitch, R., Pencharz, P., and Koren, G. (1998) "Empirical Examination of the Ability of Children to Consent to Clinical Research," *Journal of Medical Ethics*, 24(3): 158–65.

Post, S.G. (1991) "The Echo of Nuremberg: Nazi Data and Ethics," *Journal of Medical Ethics*, 17: 42–44.

Pozos, R.S. (1992) "Scientific Inquiry and Ethics: The Dachau Data," in A. Caplan (ed.) *When Medicine Went Mad: Bioethics and the Holocaust* (pp. 95–108), Totowa, NJ: Humana Press.

Pozos, R.S. and Katz, J. (1992) "The Dachau Hypothermia Study: An Ethical and Scientific Commentary," in A. Caplan (ed.) *When Medicine Went Mad: Bioethics and the Holocaust* (pp. 135–39), Totowa, NJ: Humana Press.

Rosenbaum, A.S. (1989) "The Use of Nazi Experimentation Data: Memorial or Betrayal?," *International Journal of Applied Philosophy*, 4(4): 59–67.

Rosner, F., Bennett, A.J., Cassell, E.J., Farnsworth, P., Halpern, A.L., Henry, J.B., Kanick, V., Kark, P.R., Landolt, A.B., and Loeb, L. (1991) "The Ethics of Using Scientific Data Obtained by Immoral Means," *New York State Journal of Medicine*, 91(2): 54–59.

Ross, L.F. (2003) "Do Healthy Children Deserve Greater Protection in Medical Research?," *Journal of Pediatrics*, 142: 108–12.

Rossi, W.C., Reynolds, W., and Nelson, R.M. (2003) "Child Assent and Parental Permission in Pediatric Research," *Theoretical Medicine & Bioethics*, 24(2): 131–48.

Schafer, A. (1986) "On Using Nazi Data: The Case Against," *Dialogue*, 25: 413–19.

Schonfeld T.L., Brown, J.S., Weniger, M., and Gordon, B. (2003) "Research Involving the Homeless: Arguments against Payment-in-Kind (PinK)," *IRB: Ethics & Human Research*, 25(5): 17–20.

Seidelman, W.E. (1988) "Mengele Medicus: Medicine's Nazi Heritage," *Milbank Quarterly*, 66(2): 221–39.

Sheldon, M. and Whitely, W.P. (1989) "Nazi Data: Dissociation from Evil," Commentary, *Hastings Center Report*, 19(4): 16–17.

Sterling, C.M. and Walco, G.A. (2003) "Protection of Children's Rights to Self-Determination in Research," *Ethics & Behavior*, 13(3): 237–47.

Stolberg, S.G. (2001) "Bioethicists Fall under Familiar Scrutiny," *New York Times*, August 2.

Susman, E.J., Dorn, L.D., and Fletcher, J.C. (1992) "Participation in Biomedical Research: The Consent Process as Viewed by Children, Adolescents, Young Adults, and Physicians," *Journal of Pediatrics*, 121(4): 547–52.

Tait, A.R., Voepel-Lewis, T., and Malviya S. (2003) "Do They Understand? (Part II): Assent of Children Participating in Clinical Anesthesia and Surgery Research," *Anesthesiology*, 98(3): 597–98.

Tishler, C.L. and Bartholomae, S. (2002) "The Recruitment of Normal Healthy Volunteers: A Review of the Literature on the Use of Financial Incentives," *Journal of Clinical Pharmacology*, 42: 365–75.

Tversky, A. and Kahneman, D. (1981) "The Framing of Decisions and the Psychology of Choice," *Science*, 211: 453–58.

West, D. (1998) "Radiation Experiments on Children at the Fernald and Wrentham Schools: Lessons for Protocols in Human Subject Research," *Accountability in Research*, 6(1–2): 103–25.

White, G.B. (1999) "Foresight, Insight, Oversight," *Hastings Center Report*, 29(2): 41–42.

Wilkinson, M. and Moore A. (1997) "Inducement in Research," *Bioethics*, 11(5): 373–89.

World Medical Association (1964/1975/1983/1989/1996/2000/2002) *The Declaration of Helsinki*, Online available: www.wma.net/e/policy/b3.htm (accessed September 29, 2004).

Yamagishi, K. (1997) "When a 12.86% Mortality is More Dangerous than 24.14%: Implications for Risk Communication," *Applied Cognitive Psychology*, 11: 495–506.

Yoder, L.H., O'Rourke, T.J., Etnyre, A., Spears, D.T., and Brown, T.D. (1997) "Expectations and Experiences of Patients with Cancer Participating in Phase I Clinical Trials," *Oncology Nurse Forum*, 24: 891–96.

2 Ethics of vaccine research*

Christine Grady

Vaccines are truly one of the miracles of modern science. Responsible for reducing morbidity and mortality from several formidable diseases, vaccines have made major contributions to the global public health. Generally quite safe and effective, vaccines are also an efficient and cost-effective way to prevent disease. Vaccination is the artificial introduction into the host of a preparation of a modified or synthetic antigen in order to produce a specific immune response that is able to prevent or modify disease on subsequent exposure to that antigen. Vaccines prevent infection or disease in the vaccinated individual, have an indirect protective effect on others known as herd immunity, and reduce the burden and costs of infectious diseases for society. Global eradication of the deadly disease smallpox and massive reduction in the burden of diseases like measles, mumps, polio, pertussis, diphtheria, tetanus, and several others all point to the immense value of vaccines.

Yet, despite the brilliant successes, vaccines always have been controversial. Concerns about the safety and untoward effects of vaccines, about disturbing the natural order, about compelling individuals to be vaccinated for the public good, and about the injustices of uneven access to the benefits of vaccines have been interwoven throughout the history of vaccines and remain controversial today (Macklin and Greenwood 2003; Spier 1998; Ulmer and Liu 2002). Such controversies and the scientific complexities and successes that fuel them raise significant ethical challenges in the development, public health use, and social acceptability of vaccines. This chapter will consider one aspect of these ethical challenges, those faced in the clinical testing of vaccines.

Vaccine development is a lengthy, expensive, complex, and multifaceted process of basic and clinical research, production, licensing, and marketing. Vaccines must be shown to be safe, immunogenic, and protective before they are licensed. Clinical testing in healthy human subjects is an integral and essential part of this process. After sufficient evidence of safety and desired effect is shown via *in vitro* and animal model testing, vaccine candidates are tested in human subjects in clinical trials. Carefully conducted clinical trials are an essential means of rigorously proving that a vaccine works and is safe. Without such proof unnecessary harm and expense can incur either because of lack of acceptance hindering the use of an effective vaccine or unjustified acceptance of a useless or harmful vaccine. Clinical trials of vaccines occur in progressive phases. Phase 1 studies evaluate short-term safety and immunogenicity in a small number of volunteers. Phase 2 studies expand the safety and immunogenicity evaluation and seek to determine optimal dose, schedule, and administration route in larger groups of individuals including those representative of the population that will ultimately use the vaccine. Phase 3 trials, usually randomized controlled field trials in large numbers of volunteers, seek to establish the efficacy of the vaccine candidate in preventing infection or disease.

Principles, codes, and norms of ethics guiding the ethical conduct of all clinical research apply to vaccine research; yet, most such guidance appears to focus on clinical trials of therapeutic interventions for individuals seeking treatment. Little specific attention has been given to how the ethics of vaccine trials differ.

Ethically salient features of clinical vaccine research that distinguish it from therapeutic drug research include that vaccine trials involve healthy subjects, often children, and usually (at least when testing efficacy) in very large numbers. In addition, vaccines are given not only to healthy individuals who might at some future time be exposed to the putative agent, but also to those who may never be exposed. Individuals are asked to accept some level of risk and inconvenience now for the public good and the prospect of "provisional" future individual benefit that may not be needed. Safe and effective vaccines benefit the public through reducing the burden of disease among individual members of the public, and also indirectly protecting unvaccinated members of the public through herd immunity. Individual benefit is "provisional," however, because individuals benefit directly from investigational vaccines only if they receive the active vaccine (not a placebo), the vaccine is adequately protective, and they are sufficiently exposed to the infectious agent at some future time. "In vaccine trials there are no patients, in that only a small number of vaccinees will ever become victims of the disease even if no vaccine is given" (Bjune and Gedde-Dahl 1993: 2). Unlike in drug trials where effect or lack of effect is evaluated in each individual, the desired effect in vaccine trials will be seen in a relatively small percentage of participating individuals; therefore, the number of participants in a vaccine efficacy trial must be very large. Accordingly, the risk–benefit evaluation for vaccine trials is very different than that for drug trials in that all participants accept the risk of side effects or idiosyncratic reactions to the vaccine or control justified by the potential benefit to the community.

Applying a framework for ethical research

According to a framework that synthesizes and simplifies guidance found in existing codes and regulations, seven principles are universally applicable to ethical clinical research (Emanuel *et al.* 2000). These include value, validity, fair subject selection, favorable risk–benefit ratio, independent review, informed consent, and respect for enrolled participants. Applying these principles to vaccine research allows consideration of some of the particular challenges inherent in testing vaccines (see Table 2.1).

Value

According to the ethical framework, the research question is first required to have potential social or scientific value in order to justify exposing individuals to research

Table 2.1 Framework applied to vaccine research

Elements of ethical research	Brief description	Specific considerations in vaccine research
Value	A research question that will enhance health or useful knowledge; responsive to health needs and priorities	Public health need, scientific possibility, social acceptability, political will
Validity	Appropriate and feasible design and endpoints, methodological rigor, and feasible recruitment	Endpoints and measurement of efficacy, choice of control—placebo, etc., type of randomization, feasibility of recruitment and follow up
Fair subject selection	Selection of subjects and sites based on scientific appropriateness and minimization of vulnerability and risk	Large numbers of healthy subjects, often including children. Developing country participants
Favorable risk/benefit ratio	Minimization of risks and maximization of benefits	Risks to individuals—physical, social, confidentiality, future trials. Risk of no protection. Provisional benefit to individual. Benefits to community/public good. Fair benefit evaluations
Independent review	Independent evaluation of adherence to ethical guidelines	Familiarity with vaccine research. International settings
Informed consent	Processes for providing adequate information and promoting the voluntary enrollment of subjects	Misconceptions about vaccines. Cultural and social differences, community permission
Respect for enrolled participants	Respect for and protection of subjects' rights as individuals both during and at the conclusion of research	Monitoring, right to withdraw, treatment/compensation for vaccine-induced injury

risks and inconvenience. Research that can improve health or increase useful knowledge has value. Determining the value of a vaccine trial calls for an understanding that

> the major purpose is to determine whether a vaccine is of use as a public health tool. This is in contrast to the many large scale therapeutic trials where the objective is to determine what is best for individuals. Yet, our ethical system is built around individuality . . .

> (Hall 1999: 745)

Although vaccines have significant public health value, it does not necessarily follow that every vaccine research proposal has social or scientific value. A specific vaccine study or program's value depends on its contribution to the goal of finding a safe, effective, and available vaccine useful within the context in which it will be used and acceptable to those who will use it. Clinical trials that find a vaccine not sufficiently safe or effective for widespread use can also have enormous social value. An assessment of the value of a study considers details about the public health need (e.g., the prevalence, burden, and natural history of the disease, as well as existing strategies to prevent/control it), the scientific data and possibilities (preclinical and clinical data, expected mechanism of action, immune correlates; feasibility of outcome measures); and the likely utilization of the vaccine (who will use/benefit from it, safety, cost, distribution, political will, acceptability, etc.). An important consideration is the value of the research for those participating in the vaccine testing, and how such value will be maximized through dissemination of knowledge gained, product development, availability of an effective vaccine, long-term research collaboration, and/or health system improvements.

No judgment of value is straightforward or immune from criticism, however, as illustrated by the following example in which the value of vaccine research was in dispute. A vaccine effective in preventing rotavirus infection in young children was pulled from the US market because of a high incidence of intussusception in vaccinated children. Subsequently, debates ensued about the value of proceeding with large trials planned in developing countries where disease burden and vaccine efficacy might differ. Debates highlighted differing risk/benefit calculations in developing countries where childhood deaths from rotavirus were high, as well as how acceptance of vaccine might be compromised by the US decision (Melton 2000; Weijer 2000). Assessing the value of rotavirus vaccine research was clearly, and appropriately, context dependent.

Validity

A valuable research question ethically requires a valid research design and implementation to generate useful and interpretable knowledge. Carefully chosen and rigorous study design, methodology, and implementation strategies appropriate to the research question and likely to provide interpretable generalizable data also are balanced by considerations of fairness and minimizing risk. In ensuring that the scientific design of a vaccine trial realizes social value for the primary beneficiaries, several controversial design and methodological issues can arise. Carefully defined endpoints, for example, are critical for quality science as well as ethical science. Although some vaccines prevent infection, many alter the course of infection and have their protective impact on clinical disease. In vaccine trials, surrogate endpoints can sometimes be used accurately to measure efficacy, but more often clinical endpoints are necessary. A vaccine trial evaluating clinical outcomes requires significant time, resources, and careful planning for statistical power and long-term follow-up. Furthermore, apparent conflicts can arise between the interventional care of those who become infected and the measurement of critical clinical endpoints.

For a placebo-controlled trial of an experimental vaccine against tuberculosis in Bacillus Calmette-Guerin (BCG) naïve persons, for example, a decision about purified protein derivative (PPD) testing and prophylactic treatment of those found positive had to be balanced against the need to determine the efficacy of the vaccine against clinical disease (Snider 2000). Shorter trials using surrogate endpoints to measure outcomes are attractive, but can in some cases provide misleading results.

Challenge studies in which volunteers are deliberately infected with a microbe can serve many important scientific and public health purposes, addressing questions about etiology, pathogenicity, pathogenesis, immune response, and protection (Levine 1998). Although challenge studies can be scientifically valuable and efficient, there is something disquieting about deliberately infecting research subjects, potentially causing significant discomfort in the process. Microbes amenable to challenge studies are carefully selected when the rationale is strong, the risk is low, and symptoms or effects of the challenge are self-limiting, reversible, or can be easily treated. The voluntary informed consent of the volunteer is also essential.

The choice of an appropriate control in any randomized clinical trial, including vaccine trials, can be contentious. Tension can exist between the need to ensure that the design realizes the scientific objectives while still guaranteeing research participants the health-care interventions to which they are entitled. A placebo control is acceptable when no effective vaccine is available, although it is ethically important to integrate other known preventive strategies, such as health education, into both arms of a vaccine trial. When a partially effective vaccine is available or a known effective vaccine is utilized in some places but not others, the justification for and choice of a control can be more difficult. The use of placebo controls in one arm of acellular pertussis vaccine trials conducted in Sweden and Italy, for example, was criticized despite a previous decision by the Swedish and Italian governments not to routinely use the available whole killed pertussis vaccine (Edwards and Decker 1996). These trials could not have been done in the United States where pertussis vaccine is required for children before entering school.

Randomization, a powerful research tool used to balance comparison groups, is a common feature of vaccine trials. Randomization raises ethical questions about participant autonomy, especially as empirical data show that randomization is poorly understood by research subjects (Featherstone and Donovan 1998; Leach *et al.* 1999). Although most phase 3 vaccine efficacy trials randomize individuals to demonstrate the direct protective effects of vaccine, some studies use cluster randomization or randomization by community or group. Although it can be justified by the need to evaluate herd immunity and indirect as well as direct protection from a vaccine, community or cluster randomization can jeopardize the autonomy rights of individuals within randomized communities and add further challenges to informed consent (Edwards *et al.* 1999).

Ethically, it is also necessary to ensure that a research study is feasible given the social, political, and cultural environment in which it will be conducted. In this regard, a feasible strategy for recruiting a large sample of participants and following them over time is essential, as are practical strategies for distributing and administering vaccine and for collecting and managing data. A large-scale field vaccine study in a population of migrants or nomads may not be possible, for example, or would require creative approaches for ensuring follow-up and data collection.

Fair subject selection

Fairness in subject selection is realized when subjects are chosen primarily because of their scientific appropriateness for a study, balanced by considerations of risk, benefit, and vulnerability. Fairness in the processes and outcomes of subject selection minimizes the possibility of exploiting vulnerable individuals and populations. Scientifically, those most appropriate for vaccine efficacy studies are populations with a sufficient and predictable exposure to and incidence of the disease in question to be able to show the effect of the vaccine. The sample size needed to demonstrate vaccine efficacy is usually large and calculated in part on expected disease incidence in a population, taking into account previous and evolving incidence of infection, demographics of the target population, and characteristics of those who are likely to volunteer. Historically, vaccines were often tested in "vulnerable" and captive populations, such as prisoners and the institutionalized mentally impaired. Infectious diseases were often endemic in these closed communities and conditions were easy to control. Currently, inclusion of these vulnerable groups is restricted by specific protective regulations (45CFR46, subpart C).

Considerations of who might benefit from utilization of the vaccine are important to subject selection. The Declaration of Helsinki states that "[m]edical research is only justified if there is a reasonable likelihood that the populations in which the research is carried out stand to benefit from the results of the research" (2000: paragraph 19). This has important implications when involving developing country populations in vaccine research that include not only characteristics of the disease but also likely availability and acceptability of a vaccine found to be effective.

Some have argued that phase I vaccine studies against diseases prevalent in the developing world, such as malaria or human immunodeficiency virus (HIV), should first be conducted in the country of the sponsor to minimize the possibility of exploiting vulnerable populations in resource-poor countries (Macklin and Greenwood 2003: 123). Others have argued that this requirement is not appropriate, however, since studies should be responsive to the health needs of populations, and there are good reasons to bring vaccine trials, even at early stages, to populations that will ultimately benefit the most. On the other hand, communities may still be vulnerable to exploitation if fair benefits from the research are not negotiated. (Participants in the 2001 Conference on Ethical Aspects of Research in Developing Countries 2002.)

Vaccine trials often eventually enroll large numbers of healthy children or infants, since many vaccines are ultimately used in children. The amount of research risk to which children can be exposed without corresponding benefit is limited by regulation in US-sponsored research (45CFR46, subpart D). Since children cannot protect their own interests through informed consent, parents and guardians give permission to enroll their children in vaccine research. Investigators and Institutional Review Boards (IRBs) should ensure that parents and guardians are well informed and make decisions compatible with the interests of the child. In Hepatitis A vaccine trials conducted in Northern Thailand, parents gave permission for their children to have both Hepatitis A and Hepatitis B vaccine as part of the trial in a crossover design (Innis *et al.* 1994). Parents and schoolteachers were also involved in community discussions about this trial before it began.

Risks and benefits

A favorable risk/benefit ratio exists when risks are justified by benefits to subjects and/or society and research is designed so that risks are minimized and benefits are maximized. As previously described, in vaccine research most risk accrues to individual participants, and benefits primarily to the community in finding a safe and protective vaccine. Individuals may receive future benefit from receiving an effective vaccine, but most benefit only indirectly. Both testing and use of vaccines are justified by a sort of utilitarian calculation, accepting risk of harm to a few for the benefit of many. For example, in the aforementioned Hepatitis A vaccine trial, 40,000 children were vaccinated and efficacy was determined based on 38 cases of Hepatitis A in the control group and 2 in the vaccine group. Perhaps an even clearer utilitarian justification is in place for trials involving a transmission blocking vaccine (TBV) for malaria. Individuals given only the TBV would not themselves be protected from malaria, but would interrupt the transmission cycle, protecting others in close contact with them (Hoffman and Richie 2003: 293). Infectious challenge studies involving experimental vaccines are another example of individuals accepting some risk for benefit to society and no expected benefit to themselves.

An ethical requirement of all clinical research is to minimize risk and maximize benefits. In HIV vaccine trials, for example, careful counseling and education about risk reduction strategies are a critical part of minimizing risk, as participants may incorrectly assume they are protected by an experimental vaccine and could actually increase risky behavior that exposes them to HIV.

Independent review

Through independent review, usually by an IRB or research ethics committee (REC), research is evaluated for adherence to established ethical guidelines by a committee with varied expertise and no personal or business interests in the research. There are certain issues that may make review of vaccine studies particularly challenging for review committees. Some IRBs simply lack members with expertise related to the science of vaccines and the structure of vaccine studies—for example, challenge studies or 50,000 person efficacy field trials. Similarly, as many vaccine trials involve populations in developing countries or healthy children, IRBs often will need information and sensitivity to both the context in which a study will be conducted and about current guidance and controversies in the ethics of international research and pediatric research. Review groups should make use of consultants when the expertise of their members does not meet the needs of a proposed vaccine study.

Vaccine studies that will be conducted at multiple sites also face the possible challenge of reconciling the recommendations of review groups that might not agree on details of the design or implementation of the study.

Informed consent

Once a research proposal is deemed valuable, valid, and acceptable with respect to risks, benefits, and subject selection, individuals are recruited and asked for their informed consent. Although widely valued, informed consent is imperfectly realized in much clinical research including vaccine research. In addition to possible difficulties in understanding information about the study, such as research design and procedures, risks, and possible outcomes, there are some features unique to vaccine trials that may be even more unfamiliar. Since massive public education campaigns promote the use of vaccines for public health, research participants may not appreciate how experimental vaccines in the context of research differ from standard vaccination. Two other important and common aspects of vaccine trials may be particularly hard for individuals to understand, randomization and methods for determination of vaccine efficacy. Large-scale randomized vaccine efficacy trials may randomize participants to vaccine and placebo at a 1:1 ratio. This could mean that thousands of participants in a single study will be given placebo. Studies of informed consent that have measured participant understanding in clinical trials have consistently demonstrated at best uneven comprehension of randomization and placebo design (Leach *et al.* 1999). Limited comprehension of these features of a clinical trial may be the result of both unfamiliarity with the concepts as well as misplaced therapeutic expectations or misconceptions.

Although little is known about the degree to which participants understand methods of determining vaccine efficacy, including that some participants or in a pediatric trial their children will (must) get the putative disease or infection in order to prove vaccine efficacy, it is likely to be low and surprising.

Most agree that individual informed consent is necessary for vaccine trial participation, even in circumstances when community permission is indicated (UNAIDS 2000). In certain cases, researchers may want to utilize a process of staged consent for vaccine research that may include seeking permission from community leaders, providing information to community members through group meetings, or public media, providing more detailed information to interested individuals, allowing time for deliberation, or consultation with family or health-care providers, and ultimately obtaining voluntary authorization from the person to be vaccinated (or parent/guardian). Information should be disclosed in culturally and linguistically appropriate ways. Creative strategies for educating participants about vaccine trials are often warranted especially in populations unfamiliar with research or with high rates of illiteracy.

Another debated issue is the extent to which participants in vaccine trials should be compensated for their participation. Since attitudes about compensation vary considerably, it is important to involve the community from which research participants will be recruited in establishing recruitment procedures and compensation schemes. Decisions about the appropriateness of proposed levels of compensation are often best made by the local IRB or ethics committee. However, it may be a demonstration of respect for individuals who agree to participate in vaccine research to at least cover transportation and other trial-related expenses.

When an entire community or cluster is randomized to participate in a trial of an investigational vaccine, strategies for upholding the right of individuals to refuse participation or to withdraw from the research while saving face should be sought. This may be especially important for individuals who have relatively little power or authority in their community.

Respect for enrolled participants

Research participants deserve continued respect after a study begins. Respect is demonstrated through continuous monitoring of participants' welfare, maintaining confidentiality of private information, allowing withdrawal without penalty, and assuring access to successful interventions, or new information generated by the study. Large vaccine efficacy trials often include a crossover design or other mechanism for assuring that members of the control group will receive the vaccine if it is found to be protective. Less settled are questions regarding whose responsibility it is to assure that study participants who become infected are appropriately treated. This issue was heavily debated in a series of global meetings sponsored by United Nations AIDS (UNAIDS) agency about the ethics of HIV vaccine trials, yet no consensus was reached by the time UNAIDS guidelines were published. Although most agree that vaccine trial participants who become HIV infected should receive treatment at the appropriate time, the challenge is determining how (Berkley 2003).

Providing treatment and compensation for vaccine- or research-related injuries are consistent with respect for the research participant. In the United States, the National Vaccine Injury Compensation Program provides compensation for certain injuries deemed related to licensed childhood vaccines, but no such mechanism exists for injuries sustained in clinical trials of vaccines. Liability for injury or side effects from vaccine is just one of a group of concerns cited as a disincentive for pharmaceutical industry investment in vaccine research.

Conclusion

A framework for ethical research is helpful in identifying ethical challenges common to all research as well as those unique to vaccine trials. The ethics of specific vaccine research proposals can be evaluated using the seven principles delineated here. Careful attention to ethical issues is critical to the successful development and utilization of vaccines as invaluable public health interventions.

Notes

* The views expressed here are the author's own. They do not necessarily reflect any position or policy of the National Institutes of Health, Public Health Service, or Department of Health and Human Services, and this chapter was expanded and adapted from Grady (2004).

Bibliography

Berkley, S. (2003) "Thorny Issues in the Ethics of AIDS Vaccine Trials," *Lancet*, 362: 992.

Bjune, G. and Gedde-Dahl, T.W. (1993) "Some Problems Related to Risk–Benefit Assessments in Clinical Testing of New Vaccines," *Institutional Review Board*, 15(1): 1–5.

Edwards, K. and Decker, M. (1996) "Acellular Pertussis Vaccine for Infants," *New England Journal of Medicine*, 334(6): 391–92.

Edwards, S., Braunholtz, D., Lilford, R., and Stevens, A. (1999) "Ethical Issues in the Design and Conduct of Cluster Randomized Controlled Trials," *British Medical Journal*, 318: 1407–09.

Emanuel, E., Wendler, D., and Grady, C. (2000) "What Makes Clinical Research Ethical?," *Journal of American Medical Association*, 283(20): 2701–11.

Featherstone, K. and Donovan, J. (1998) "Random Allocation or Allocation at Random? Patients' Perspectives of Participation in a Randomized Controlled Trial," *British Medical Journal*, 317: 1177–80.

Grady, C. (2004) "Ethics of Vaccine Research," *Nature Immunology*, 5(5): 465–68.

Hall, A.J. (1999) "Vaccine Trials and Ethics," *International Journal of Tuberculosis and Lung Disease*, 3(9): 745–46.

Hoffman, S. and Richie, T. (2003) "Disease States and Vaccines: Malaria," in B. Bloom and P. Lambert (eds) *The Vaccine Book* (pp. 291–310), San Diego, CA: Elsevier Science USA.

Innis, B.L., Snitbhan, R., Kunasol, P., Laorakpongse, T., Poopatanakool, W., Kozik, C.A., Suntayakorn, S., Suknuntapong, T., Safary, A., Tang, D.B., and Boslego, J.W. (1994) "Protection against Hepatitis A by an Inactivated Vaccine," *Journal of American Medical Association*, 271(17): 1328–34.

Leach, A., Hilton, S., Greenwood, B., Manneh, E., Dibba, B., Wilkins, A., and Mulholland, E. (1999) "An Evaluation of the Informed Consent Process during a Trial of *Haemophilus Influenza* Type B Conjugate Vaccine Undertaken in the Gambia, West Africa," *Social Science and Medicine*, 48: 139–49.

Levine, M.M. (1998) "Experimental Challenge Studies in the Development of Vaccines for Infectious Diseases," in S. Plotkin, F. Brown, and F. Horaud (eds) *Preclinical and Clinical Development of New Vaccines, Development of Specifications for Biotechnology Pharmaceutical Products*, 95 (pp. 169–74), Basel: Karger.

Macklin, R. and Greenwood, B. (2003) "Ethics and Vaccines," in B. Bloom and P. Lambert (eds) *The Vaccine Book* (pp. 119–27), San Diego, CA: Elsevier Science USA.

Melton, L. (2000) "Lifesaving Vaccine Caught in an Ethical Minefield," *Lancet*, 356: 318.

Participants in the 2001 Conference on Ethical Aspects of Research in Developing Countries (2002) "Ethics: Fair Benefits for Research in Developing Countries," *Science*, 298: 2133–34.

Snider, D.E. (2000) "Ethical Issues in Tuberculosis Vaccine Trials," *Clinical Infectious Diseases*, 30(Suppl 3): S271–75.

Spier, R.E. (1998) "Ethical Aspects of Vaccines and Vaccination," *Vaccine*, 16(19): 1788–94.

Ulmer, J.B. and Liu, M. (2002) "Ethical Issues for Vaccines and Immunization," *Nature Reviews Immunology*, 2: 291–94.

UNAIDS (2000) *Ethical Considerations in HIV Preventive Vaccines*, Geneva, Switzerland: UNAIDS.

Weijer, C. (2000) "The Future of Research into Rotavirus Vaccine," *British Medical Journal*, 321: 525–26.

World Medical Association (WMA) (2000) "Declaration of Helsinki: Ethical Principles for Medical Research Involving Human Subjects," Online available: http://www.wma.net/e/policy/b3.htm (accessed November 18, 2004).

3   Ethical issues in the conduct of genetic research

Lisa S. Parker and Lauren Matukaitis Broyles

At the inception of the Human Genome Project (HGP), ethical attention centered primarily on the implications of genetic research, not its conduct. Concern focused on the ways that genetic findings might be (mis)used by individuals and social institutions (e.g., insurers, employers, courts). The primary risks of research participation were deemed to be the psychosocial risks of learning genetic information about oneself or the possibility that third parties would obtain access to the information. Because of the nature of genetic information, not only individuals but also families and groups bear these risks, the magnitude of which remains largely unknown. The section on genetic research in the *IRB Guidebook* published in 1993 by the Office for Human Research Protections (OHRP) (formerly the Office for the Protection from Research Risks (OPRR)) focused on how to address these psychosocial risks of individual and group harm within existing guidelines, regulations (45 CFR 46), and ethical frameworks (e.g., informed consent). Scientists were largely trusted with the ethical conduct of research.

After over a decade, the issues outlined in the *Guidebook* remain salient. There is greater awareness, however, that the design and conduct of genetic research present challenges for investigators and regulators, prompting efforts to revise the *Guidebook*, just as post-research use of genetic findings prompted public discussion, institutional change, and in some cases, legislation. In particular, the revised *Guidebook* (2005) is expected to pay greater attention to concerns about the procurement, banking, and analysis of biological materials; group harms and community consultation; and informed consent issues, especially in pedigree studies.

It would, however, be as misleading to engage in genetic exceptionalism about genetic research as it is to treat genetic information as different in kind from other health information. Most ethical issues substantially overlap with those in other research arenas featured in this volume because the field of genetic research comprises benchwork, animal modeling, epidemiological studies, statistical/computational research, and clinical trials. Even discussion of community consultation for genetic research has its roots in requirements for such consultation for research on emergency interventions (e.g., resuscitation research). As in other research arenas, issues attach to every stage of a particular project—protocol development, recruitment and enrollment of subjects, data collection and analysis, and dissemination of results.

Even though most types of genetic research share basic ethical considerations, some arise more acutely with respect to particular types of genetic research, from projects seeking to identify patterns of inheritance and then specific genes, to those testing for genetic mutations, to gene transfer research. This chapter considers issues in the contexts where they arise most acutely or present unusual challenges to existing ethical and regulatory frameworks.

Pedigrees and positional cloning: human subjects, recruitment and enrollment, and informed consent

Pedigree studies are employed to identify patterns of inheritance, and then pedigrees are used in linkage studies to identify specific genes, or the link between particular genetic mutations and conditions of interest. Informed consent to such studies is complicated by practical and conceptual problems (Beskow *et al.* 2004). It is difficult to assess and disclose the risks and benefits of participation because of both their psychosocial nature, and a lack of data on the actual magnitude of risks of stigma and discrimination, as well as the likelihood and source of privacy breach, especially given the familial nature of genetic information. The right of subjects to withdraw from pedigree studies must be explained carefully: information that has already been used in pedigree or DNA analysis cannot be removed and the data reanalyzed without it, although individuals may have their information removed from the pedigree (the "family tree" that is one of the tangible products of pedigree research), and their DNA sample may be analyzed no further and should be destroyed. Moreover, given that the family is the unit of study, concern has been raised about intrafamilial pressures to participate in pedigree studies, although such pressures are neither likely to be greater than those normally exerted by family members on each other nor are they likely to violate standards of voluntariness for informed consent (Parker and Lidz 1994). Finally, in addition to raising concerns about group harms (discussed in the section on group harms, community consultation, and consent), pedigree studies present vexing conceptual questions about what constitutes private information, research data, minimal risk, and the status of being a human subject of research.

In conducting genetic pedigree studies, family medical history information is typically obtained from an affected individual ("proband") first to identify families that may be relevant for study, and next to identify members within a family who may be relevant to the research. The 1993 *Guidebook* comments, "The ethical question presented by this practice is whether that information can become part of the study without the consent of the person about whom the data pertains. While no consensus on this issue has yet been reached, Institutional Review Boards (IRBs) may consider collection of data in this manner acceptable, depending on the nature of the risks and sensitivities involved" (OPRR 1993: 5–46). Thus, a tentative pedigree has typically been constructed with information supplied by a proband, because it is often impossible to determine the eligibility of a particular family without knowing the relationship among affected members. During the first decade of the HGP, concern about protecting privacy and confidentiality in pedigree studies centered first on the privacy of the proband, and subsequently on protecting intrafamilial confidentiality of other family members.

Investigation of a nongenetic survey study at Virginia Commonwealth University (VCU), in 1999, led the OPRR to (re)interpret informed consent requirements for human subject research to apply to all living persons about whom the researcher gathers identifiable private information, including family members mentioned in a family history by a proband. Although of particular interest for the conduct of genetic pedigree studies, this interpretation is equally salient for any research that involves obtaining information about third parties from those specifically enrolled as research subjects. In the VCU study, the father of an enrolled adult subject believed that her responses to some survey questions would violate his or their family's privacy. Preserving the division of labor and authority between the federal regulatory level and local IRBs, the OPRR faulted the VCU IRB for failing *to consider* whether informed consent was required from those family members about whom information was collected; OPRR did not (pre)judge the question itself. Conservative IRBs, however, may interpret the OPRR to have found merit in the father's concerns, and require that investigators either seek informed consent from similarly situated third parties (sometimes called "secondary subjects"), or seek formal IRB waiver of the consent requirement. In response, the American Society of Human Genetics published a statement entitled "Should family members about whom you collect only medical history information for your research be considered 'human subjects'?" that opines:

> If, in large family studies, each family member must be enrolled as a "human subject", with informed consent procedures, before any medical information about them can be collected, obtaining family histories will be enormously cumbersome and prohibitive, and will seriously impede medical research. Unless a "waiver" is granted, the project may no longer be feasible.
>
> (2000)

Genetic pedigree studies proceed in stages, beginning with the sketch of a tentative pedigree to identify families of research interest on the basis of unverified, and usually nonexpert or "hearsay" information of the proband. An interpretation of informed consent requirements that would prohibit collection of such information at this initial stage without the express (and written) consent of the family members about whom the proband would be providing information creates an apparent "catch 22." How can investigators obtain consent to obtain information about family members without first obtaining information about them in order to contact them? In fact, investigators might supply probands with a postage-paid "initial contact letter" for each family member. This letter would ask the relative to consent to be contacted by the investigator by returning a "response letter" granting permission. The investigator will then ask some questions about the individual's medical history and obtain permission to recontact the relative to enroll her/him in the study, if the family proves eligible. Some argue that in addition to being costly and likely reducing recruitment rates, such a process of seeking informed consent from family members at this initial stage of research would actually multiply the opportunities for breach of their privacy and increase the psychosocial risks associated with pedigree study participation (and even nonparticipation) (Parker 2002). Except for the well-publicized VCU case, there is little documentation of family members' discomfort with previously employed procedures for initiating pedigree studies. Research is needed to explore different methods of recruiting family members in pedigree studies, with data collected on their privacy concerns, the effect of different contact methods on rates and costs of recruitment, the magnitude of anxiety imposed by different methods (on members of both unaffected and affected branches of families), and the frequency of other negative sequelae (e.g., self-stigmatization, social stigma, and discrimination). Even a paternalistic practice like human subject protection should be responsive to the actual preferences of those it seeks to protect.

The requirement of informed consent would not apply if the information obtained were either not private or not individually identifiable (45 CFR 46.102(f)), or if information gathering activities at the stage of determining eligibility for study were specifically classified as not constituting research, and thus those reported on by the proband were specifically considered not to be human subjects. Guidance from the OHRP is, however, usually interpreted by IRBs to encompass information gathering at this early stage as research development subject to informed consent requirements (2004). However, IRBs are permitted to grant a *waiver* of the requirement for written informed consent if four conditions are met: (1) the research involves no more than minimal risk to subjects; (2) the waiver will not adversely affect subjects' rights and welfare; (3) the research could not practicably be carried out without the waiver; and (4) whenever appropriate, after participation, subjects will be provided with additional pertinent information (45 CFR 46.116(d)). In the absence of changes in the Common Rule's characterization of human subjects or what it means to "obtain" private identifiable information, some argue that granting of such a waiver may be the best way to proceed because most genetic pedigree research meets the conditions for waiver for this initial stage of study (Parker 2002). One commentator appears to disagree, especially with respect to research on "conditions with a behavioral or psychiatric component" or possibly stigmatizing personal traits, such as sexual orientation or reproductive history, commenting:

> It may be appropriate for an IRB to consider protocols to be greater than minimal risk for secondary subjects [individuals about whom a proband reports information] when the family history pursued includes such highly sensitive information. In contrast, IRBs may consider protocols to be of less than minimal risk when the family history includes only information about existing health conditions or low or moderate sensitivity, such as heart disease, cancer, or diabetes, and when strong data security measures are in place.
>
> (Botkin 2001: 201)

The observation that behavioral and psychiatric conditions are more stigmatizing than other common illnesses is, unfortunately, quite accurate, although treating research on them differently from other research may contribute to their exceptional status.

Moreover, pedigree studies do not merely gather existing health information, which might present relatively low risks, but instead may generate new health information by identifying individuals (and branches of families) as being at risk for disease (Botkin 2001). Beginning with a proband (e.g., someone with breast cancer), a pedigree study involves identifying other affected relatives and their relationship, thereby revealing the inheritance pattern of the condition (e.g., autosomal dominant inheritance of BRCA1/2 breast cancer mutations). With the collection of DNA samples from family members and gene mapping techniques, it is possible to identify the gene (or genes) associated with the condition despite incomplete understanding of its biochemical basis. Thus, it is possible to learn a great deal about family relationships and individual members' risk of inheriting (or having already inherited) particular genes without learning much about how to treat the condition (as with Huntington disease (HD)), or even the likelihood of the condition becoming manifest in a particular at-risk individual (a function of the gene's penetrance), or its severity (a function of the gene's variable expression). For that reason, participation in any genetic pedigree research—whether on stigmatizing conditions or not—poses more than minimal risk, and informed consent is required (Merz 1996).

Some individuals would prefer not to know whether they are at increased risk for developing a particular condition. The values of well-being and autonomy that generally support one's right to know information relevant to one's health also support one's right to choose not to know it. Such information may result in disrupted family relationships, anxiety, a sense of "survivor's guilt" among those not at increased risk, changed self-image, and if the information becomes known to others, stigma (e.g., being viewed as "unmarriageable" or tainted), or risks related to employment or insurability. In addition to being associated with genetic findings, these psychosocial sequelae may result from incidental findings—information learned, but not specifically sought, in the course of genetic research (e.g., misattributed paternity or risk of other health-related conditions). Because of these risks and because of individuals' autonomous interests in choosing whether or not to contribute to scientific research, subjects must be asked for their informed consent to participate. Therefore, although consent requirements may be waived at the stage of identifying families for study, when a pedigree study is actually being conducted, with the collection and analysis of health information, family relationships, and in some cases, DNA samples, informed consent must be obtained from those represented on the pedigree. Finally, because of the familial nature of genetic information, some negative sequelae may attach to family membership, even though one obtains no specific genetic information oneself. Individual informed consent is inadequate to protect from these group harms that may affect families and communities (e.g., stigmatization of Ashkenazi Jewish women because of a breast cancer-related founder effect in that population). These issues are discussed later.

Procurement, storage, and analysis of biological materials

The procurement, banking, and use of human biological materials (HBMs) for DNA analysis also raise questions about the applicability of human subjects protections and informed consent requirements. While some HBM are indeed explicitly donated for research—either for a specific research project or for more or less unspecified future research purposes—many samples in repositories are merely leftover from clinical diagnostic and therapeutic interventions. Their use in research may not have been contemplated by those who once housed the materials. Therefore, there is a need to develop policies not only to govern prospectively the procurement of HBM for research, but also to manage ethically repositories of existing samples.

President Clinton's National Bioethics Advisory Commission (NBAC) and several working groups—for example, of the National Institutes of Health (NIH), Centers for Disease Control and Prevention, American College of Medical Genetics, and American Society for Human Genetics—have considered these issues and offer guidance, although no clear consensus has emerged (American College of Medical Genetics 1995; American Society of Human Genetics 1996; Clayton *et al.* 1995; NBAC 1999). The most detailed guidance document, from the NBAC, categorizes HBM depending on the likelihood that the initial human source may be identified; see Table 3.1 (1999).

The appropriate guidelines for using stored tissue samples depend very much on whether private identifiable information is associated with the sample, and on who has legitimate access to that information, as well as the likelihood that a third party may obtain illicit access. Because of the value of being able to link genetic mutations with clinical conditions, de-identified but coded samples are frequently used in genetic research to preserve the link between sample and clinical information. Consider, for example, that having learned through pedigree and positional cloning

Table 3.1 Categories of HBM

Repository collections	*Research samples*
Unidentified specimens: specimens for which identifiable personal information was never collected or maintained by the repository and therefore cannot be retrieved	*Unidentified samples*: "anonymous" samples supplied by repositories to researchers from a collection of unidentified human specimens
Identified specimens: specimens linked to personal identifiable information allowing the identification of the human source by name, patient number, or clear pedigree location	*Unlinked samples*: "anonymized" samples lacking identifiers or codes which could link an individual sample to a particular human being
	Coded samples: "de-identified"/"linked"/ "identifiable" samples provided by repositories to researchers from specimens labeled with a code as opposed to identifying information such as name or social security number
	Identified samples: samples provided by repositories labeled with identifying information such as name or social security number

studies that mutations at the BRCA1/2 loci on chromosomes 17 and 13, respectively, are associated with increased breast cancer risk, genetic researchers might want to test stored breast tumor samples or blood samples in a large repository to determine what percentage of those breast cancers may be associated with the newly identified BRCA1/2 genes, or how many different mutations at those loci may be discovered. Using stored HBM rather than recruiting newly diagnosed breast cancer patients for such a study may save considerable time and money, as well as reduce burden on those patients. On the other hand, some patients whose tumor biopsies were previously stored may not have consented to their use in research. Others may have known about the banking of their HBM and even consented to its use in research, but never envisioned that they might be used in *genetic* research. In decades past, cancer was not viewed as a genetic condition by the public, which generally thought of cancer research as focused solely on cure or treatment, not on risk assessment and prevention. A fundamental question is whether informed consent for the research use of stored HBM is required, and the degree to which "blanket" consents or consent for nonspecified research purposes fulfill informed consent requirements, or at least their ethical spirit, if not the letter of regulatory requirements.

Some investigators and IRBs argue that because, under an appropriately designed protocol, the identity of the sample sources is not known to, or even knowable by, researchers (but only by those managing the repository of existing specimens), such research should be exempt from federal regulations governing human subjects research, the "Common Rule" (45 CFR 46.101(b)(4)). Moreover, some argue that because investigators neither interact with subjects nor have identifiable private information about them, research on stored HBM should not be considered human subjects research (45 CFR 46.102(f)). Nevertheless, NBAC recommendations suggest that research with coded samples should be considered human subjects research and thus subject to Common Rule protections, although waiver of consent requirements may be considered by IRBs. The OHRP has provided specific guidance on these issues (2004). Research utilizing unidentified samples (or samples from those who are deceased) is not deemed to be human subjects research; however, according to NBAC, research with unlinked/anonymized samples should be considered human subjects research, although it is likely to qualify for exemption from IRB review (1999).

Because of the possible harms of linking individuals to results of research on their HBM, protection of individuals' privacy is key. Devising appropriate protocols to separate individuals' identifying information from their samples and associated clinical information (e.g., health status, age of onset of condition, demographic information), securely storing data and samples, and considering application for a Federal Certificate of Confidentiality are privacy protection measures incumbent upon repositories and/or research teams. Requiring informed consent to the procurement, storage, and future use of HBM affords additional privacy protection by ensuring individuals the right to refuse to participate.

The process of obtaining consent to this banking for research purposes should be separate from the consent process for any therapeutic or diagnostic intervention (e.g., surgical biopsy) that results in the sample itself. The NBAC recommends that individuals be offered a variety of choices about future use of samples, the degree of identifiability they accept, and the degree to which they are willing to be recontacted for additional information or consent for use of samples in future research (1999). Subjects' right to withdraw their HBM from repositories (or a particular study) must be carefully explained. Although their samples may be withdrawn and destroyed, along with any associated clinical information, data gleaned from previous analysis of those samples cannot be withdrawn. Informed consent to specific studies employing HBM would involve disclosure of the nature and aim of the research, the possibility that the research may lead to the development of commercially valuable products like diagnostic tests (subjects are usually informed that they retain no financial interests), and the duration, storage, and possibility of future use of the HBM (Clayton *et al.* 1995). Individuals would be asked to grant permission for such future use or to agree to be recontacted to obtain such permission or additional health-related information (American College of Medical Genetics 1995). There is clear consensus that individuals should be asked to give informed consent to the procurement and banking of HBM for research purposes; however, for several reasons, obtaining informed consent for specific projects involving stored HBM is challenging, and no consensus has emerged about how to proceed.

Research using stored HBM raises two sets of questions. The first set focuses on whether the proposed study qualifies for a waiver of consent. The criteria for granting a waiver were outlined above. Two issues to be considered prior to granting a waiver of consent are discussed in detail in subsequent sections. These are, first, consideration of whether the study will investigate traits with political, cultural, or economic significance for subjects, and whether the protocol could negatively affect the subject's socially identifiable community; second, the requirement of a plan for disclosure of "relevant findings" to individuals or their providers, if the situation warrants. Here, the primary question is whether the use of stored HBM presents no more than minimal risk to contributors of the samples. Research use of de-identified samples probably presents a lower risk of privacy breach than is incurred in routine clinical care (Parker 2002); however, some have argued that research on stored HBM should not be routinely classed as minimal risk (American Society of Human Genetics 1996; Merz 1996), and the NBAC report advocates evaluating such risks directly, rather than in comparison to the sometimes inadequate privacy protection practices found in clinical settings. How likely is it that subjects will be identified, who is likely to do so, and how great would be the harms of identification? In the presence of adequate protocols to de-identify samples, to protect the codes from being illicitly "cracked," and to prevent the inadvertent release of information to third parties, the risks are likely to be minimal.

Of course, informed consent is supposed to protect not only welfare interests, but also interests in self-determination. A waiver of the consent requirement will contravene individuals' rights not to contribute to the conduct of the study. Therefore, the justification for ignoring this right must be substantial. Such justification is usually thought to lie in the combination of the scientific benefit of pursuing the research questions and the impossibility of conducting the study if the consent requirement were imposed; however, this justification involves at least minimal sacrifice of individual rights for the social good (Woodward 1999). Moreover, there is considerable ambiguity in the notion of research being "impossible" to conduct if consent were required. Increased expense of obtaining informed consent is not considered to render the research relevantly impossible, even if in practical terms, the research would not be funded at that level. In most cases, the research could not be conducted within the same timeframe or with the same pool of samples, but, the same or very similar research question could be pursued with a pool of prospectively collected samples from consenting subjects. Public discussion and research on the preferences of past and prospective HBM donors should be conducted to determine whether people are generally willing to have stored samples used for research without further opportunities to consent or refuse. It may be that what people most care about is the protection of the privacy of their health information; however, it is also possible that a substantial number want to control their contribution to research or to know that they have made an altruistic contribution.

The second set of questions about using stored HBM arises when waiver of the informed consent requirement is not justifiable, or when informed consent for some future use has been obtained, but there is a question regarding whether a proposed study falls within the scope of the permission granted. Initial informed consent documents corresponding to repository samples of HBM should be provided by investigators during IRB review in order for the IRB to determine their applicability to the current investigation; however, documents may or may not indicate the individuals' preferences about future use of such samples. Of course, when preferences are indicated, investigators should respect them. Individuals may refuse sample use in any future research; may request that their samples be used only in research on disorders or diseases which represent their interests; may refuse their samples' use for research on potentially stigmatizing conditions (e.g., substance use or psychiatric illness); may decline use by commercial entities; or may consider long-term storage to violate cultural or religious beliefs (Clayton *et al.* 1995).

Suppose that, as is in fact true, many breast cancer patients gave informed consent to the retention of their tumor biopsies for "use in future research." Would every research question qualify for access to those stored samples? While research on breast cancer would seem to be covered, and perhaps research on other cancers would similarly be included, some might argue that use of those samples for research on the genetic basis of sexual orientation should be conducted only with specific (re)consent. It is indeed unlikely that women contemplated such a research question in, for example, the 1980s when they had their cancer surgeries, years before a link between breast cancer risk and "lesbian lifestyle" was alleged. The "catch 22" illustrated by this example is that recontacting these patients, either for permission to use their samples or for information about their sexual orientation, may also be perceived as an invasion of their privacy. Even if the recontact did not concern the sensitive topic of sexual orientation, but merely sought permission to use their samples in research on diabetes or heart disease, the question might prompt anxiety about other health risks or rekindle memories of their cancer experience. There is no clearly best solution to this dilemma. The best guide, however, is that future or secondary uses of HBM that most closely resemble the original or specifically contemplated use may most justifiably be undertaken without recontacting for specific consent. Contact that is closest in time to the original consent to banking, and thus the least "out of the blue" may be thought to be least intrusive. Those who agreed to some research use or to some degree of recontact may be thought to be most receptive to being recontacted for additional information or permission to use samples. These rules of thumb could be investigated, and data about subjects' responses should be collected in actual instances of recontact/reconsent.

Disclosure of interim results and incidental findings to subjects

Although the goal of all genetic research is generalizable knowledge, many types of genetic research may yield information about individual subjects—for example, inadvertent information about their family relationships or health status, or about their risk for the disease under study, particularly whether they carry a specific genetic mutation. Should this information be disclosed to subjects? On this issue, like many others in this chapter, it is wise to practice preventive ethics (Forrow *et al.* 1993; Parker 1994). In other words, just as patterns of illness may be noted, medical problems anticipated, and preventive medical interventions designed, investigators may note and anticipate recurrent ethical problems and devise means of preventing them. Practicing preventive ethics about the disclosure of research results and incidental findings would dictate that investigators state up front in the informed consent process whether such information will or will not be disclosed.

Taking family histories for pedigree studies or genetic testing for linkage analysis, just like prenatal testing in a clinical context, may be anticipated to reveal cases of misattributed paternity and adoption. There is no reason to reveal such incidental findings, although subjects should be warned during the informed consent process that the publication of a pedigree or increased general knowledge about the family's condition of interest may enable relatives to decipher such information about each other. Sometimes diagnostic tests or clinical examinations used to confirm subjects' health status may reveal conditions of which the subjects are unaware. Subjects must be informed during informed consent whether referrals for appropriate clinical care will be made. Diagnosis, in the research context, of suicidal ideation or of other immediate life-threatening conditions should trigger referral for immediate clinical care; however, discovery of other health conditions need not, so long as subjects know that the testing and examination undertaken through the research protocol should not be relied upon for their health care, as no "feedback loop" of (nonemergency) health information to them is planned. Indeed, referrals for care as a result of such examinations in the research context may exacerbate the therapeutic misconception that plagues all research by blurring the research–therapy distinction (Appelbaum *et al.* 1982).

For a variety of reasons, it is generally best to implement a policy of nondisclosure with respect to research results. Because not only the risks, but also the benefits of knowing genetic information are mediated by personal and social circumstances, as well as personal values and beliefs, it is difficult to argue that imposing information on an individual—acting on a perceived "duty to disclose"—could be justified by potential benefit to the recipient. Only in the rare case that the individual could use the information to prevent very probable, very serious harm might investigators justify violating an individual's putative right not to know—for example, in the case of hemochromatosis, in which overabsorbtion of iron leads to liver damage, or myotonic dystrophy, which presents particular hazards of anesthesia management (Buchanan 1998).

The more likely case, however, is one in which a subject *asks* for research results, for example, of a direct genetic test or linkage analysis, especially when such information is not accessible through testing outside of a research protocol. During linkage studies to identify breast cancer genes, some subjects sought "interim results"—that is, they wanted to know whether their particular DNA profile was being linked to the genetic mutation emerging as one associated with breast cancer in their families—in order to help plan prophylactic mastectomies. One problem with the premature disclosure of such information is that the enrollment of additional subjects and acquisition of additional information may reverse the indication, changing one's status from "increased risk" to near "general population risk." Like those who conduct clinical trials or any study that generates information of relevance to people's decision-making, genetic researchers must establish justified endpoints for their studies and appropriate stopping rules. Departures from such protocols for the general termination of the study because a hypothesis has been confirmed, to instead offer individual disclosures, are extremely difficult to justify. The NBAC suggests that disclosure be construed as "an exceptional circumstance" (1999). Additionally, the NBAC recommends that disclosure be made only when three criteria are fully met: the findings must be scientifically valid and confirmed, they must pose significant health implications for the subject, and treatment for these implications must be readily available. Again, if there is reason to continue the study, it is unlikely that interim results meet the standards of scientific validity. Moreover, according to federal regulations, only results of testing conducted in specially certified laboratories may be reported for the purpose of "diagnosis, prevention, or treatment of any disease . . . or the health assessment of individual patients" (Clinical Laboratory Improvement Amendments of 1988, 42 CFR 494.3(b)(2)). In addition, few research teams have adequate personnel or funding to provide appropriate genetic counseling. If genetic information is disclosed to subjects, they should be referred for such counseling.

Some authors point out that the question of disclosure of genetic or other health information also raises the question of the potential liability to researchers. If relevant diagnostic or therapeutic interventions become available, and researchers fail to notify subjects, could they be held legally liable for subsequent harm to the individual? The question of whether clinicians have a duty, or even a right, to contact patients (or their relatives) to disclose genetic risks to them is one on which there is no clear consensus (*Pate v. Threlkel* 1995; *Safer v. Pack* 1996). Such liability, however, is deemed a minor risk for researchers, especially if they inform subjects of the limits of disclosure during the informed consent process (Clayton *et al.* 1995).

Group harms, community consultation, and consent

Two factors persistently complicate assessment of the risks and benefits of genetic research, and thus the processes of recruitment and informed consent. First, not only individuals, but also a group as a whole—for example, a family or an ethnic or a geographic group—may be harmed (or benefited) by genetic information. Second, even individuals who have not participated in research and who have not learned genetic information about themselves may be subjected to harms (and in some cases, benefits), in virtue of their membership in groups or the social identity ascribed to them by others. The first type of risk is borne by the group or community itself, while the second is borne by the individual but in virtue of his/her membership in the group. The two types of risk are distinct, and the distinction relates to the different commitments of communitarianism and liberal individualism; the possibility that communities as a whole may be harmed by genetic research assumes that communities themselves have interests distinct from the interests of their members. Indeed, some propose addition of "respect for communities" as a fourth moral principle to the three principles articulated in *The Belmont Report*—respect for persons, beneficence, and justice—to grant moral status to interests of the community, interests which may or may not be in conflict with those of the individual (Weijer 1999).

In practice, the two types of risk often manifest simultaneously and similarly. The effects of discrimination against linguistic minorities, for example, are borne by individual speakers of the language, as well as by the community that would otherwise have a more freely flourishing linguistically distinct culture (ex hypothesi something in the community's interest). Thus, measures that would enhance the protection of putative community interests may also protect individuals from harms resulting from ascribed group identity. These risks arise in genetic research because genetic information is familial, and because some populations have higher prevalence of some conditions than others, perhaps because of a higher frequency of a genetic mutation in some populations due to the mutation's presence in ancestors and subsequent breeding patterns (a "founder effect").

With respect to various ethnic, religious, geographic, and cultural groups, as well as families, genetic research raises concerns about group stigmatization and discrimination (Foster *et al.* 1997/1998; Weijer 1999), decisions to enroll in research (Davis 2000), collective privacy (Foster and Freeman 1998), and profitable opportunities (Clayton 2002; National Research Council (NRC) 1997). Most significantly, groups or families, and their members, may be labeled as "defective," "inferior," or "tainted," and face subsequent social, economic, or political discrimination. Some communities may fear being "guinea pigs" for genetic research, feel exploited by researchers' methods and approaches, or perceive little benefit to their group as a whole. Finally, communities may have concerns related to potential economic interests of the researchers or others, including the financial and symbolic implications of patenting genetic material, as well as concern about what compensation the community may receive for participation (Clayton 2002; Foster and Freeman 1998; NRC 1997). Given historical examples of discriminatory practices and policies carried out based on genetic information or its misinterpretation, these concerns are warranted

(Andrews 1997; Bradby 1996). Therefore, genetic research challenges the assumption that, together with adherence to other regulatory safeguards, individual informed consent is sufficient to warrant participation and to protect human subjects (Mitchell and Happe 2001; Weber and Bissell 2002). Community consultation and community consent are proposed to supplement, not supplant, the process of individual informed consent.

The primary goal of community consultation is the creation of a partnership to protect the multiple interests of the community members, including their collective identity, which may be affected by research and the dissemination of results. Community consultation is ideally conceptualized as an ongoing dialogue between the researchers and community throughout all phases of the research process, from formulation of the research question and protocol development through publication and dissemination of research results (Weijer and Emanuel 2000). It may be implemented through the use of focus groups, open houses, town meetings, telephone contacts, or other dialogue between the research team and the community from which subjects are sought. Several authors have detailed guidelines for implementing community consultation protocols (Foster *et al.* 1998; Weijer 1999; Weijer and Emanuel 2000; Weijer *et al.* 1999). In determining the need for community consultation, investigators should consider the research's potential negative effect on the community, especially in light of its past experiences, unique traditions and practices, and social structure (NIH 2002a). Though not currently required for federally funded genetic studies or by most IRBs, community consultation can benefit both the community and researchers by evidencing researchers' respect for potential subjects, allowing community members to raise questions and concerns about risk and benefit, prospectively creating a forum to address issues surrounding study outcomes, and enhancing the public's scientific literacy by dispelling common myths about the promise and potential of genetic research. Community consultation can also uncover weaknesses in study design that might undermine the study's feasibility or the validity and generalizability of its outcomes, provide information to improve recruitment strategies and the informed consent process, and provide the foundation for an appropriately trusting relationship that facilitates the entire research process (NIH 2002a).

Despite these obvious benefits, the idea of community consultation has been criticized on conceptual and pragmatic grounds, including its limited feasibility for large, diverse communities, as well as its added cost and burden to researchers (Mitchell and Happe 2001; Reilly 1998). Furthermore, concerns about inherent paternalism, including the substitution of community representatives' judgments for those of individual members, and the risk of investigators' "forum shopping" for the population with which it is easiest to work, raise justice-oriented concerns about community consultation (Reilly 1998: 698). Conceptual concerns begin with the difficulty of defining the relevant community and of justly determining who may speak for, or make decisions on behalf of, the community and its members. Communities are rarely homogeneous with respect to their members' beliefs, goals, and values (Davis 2000), and degrees of human connectedness are dynamic as social structures evolve (Weijer and Emanuel 2000). Identifying the community spokesperson or decision-maker may also be difficult, especially in the context of large or diverse communities. Had, for example, community consultation been implemented prior to the institution of sickle cell screening in the United States, who would or should have spoken for the diverse population of African Americans? Ensuring that all viewpoints within the community are represented may be difficult, or impossible, thereby raising concern about which standpoints within the community receive the greatest attention and privilege (Davis 2000).

Membership in a community may be based on a variety of characteristics, including shared experience of a health-related condition (Davis 2000; Weijer and Emanuel 2000); see Table 3.2. It must also be recognized, however, that possession of these characteristics does not necessitate community membership or self-identification. Someone with Ashkenazi Jewish genetic heritage, for example, may have no affiliation or identification with this group, its values, or goals. While this individual may be of interest to a genetic researcher studying this population, the person may have few (or different) concerns to raise in a community consultation process (Davis 2000). At the same time, upon dissemination of results of genetic research in this population, such an individual may suffer harms, like stigma, in virtue of others' ascription of this group identity to her. She may also benefit from the group-related genetic information (e.g., by seeking increased mammographic screening or even genetic testing), or suffer harm from it (e.g., increased anxiety). Consulting with representatives of "the Ashkenazi Jewish community" may mitigate, but not entirely avoid, some of the harms to which such an individual may be subject.

Many concerns about community consultation extend to the related but distinct notion of community *consent*. Community consent involves the community's provision of formal, informed permission for the research to proceed. Community consent may arise from, but is not the same as, community consultation. With the exception of sovereign First Nations within North America, community consent is neither required by federal regulations nor considered to be practical, nor is it considered even desirable by those who emphasize liberal over communitarian values, or the rights of individuals over the interests of communities. Research involving First Nations, however, typically requires the approval of tribal leaders and IRBs (NIH 2002a; NRC 1997). Where community consent is applicable, it can be viewed as supplementary to, but never a substitute for, individual consent to participation

Table 3.2 Characteristics constituting community or group identity

Type of group identity	Examples
Genetic	Possessing genes associated with Ashkenazi Jews
Ethnic or cultural	Being Ashkenazi Jewish, speaking Polish
Religious	Membership in the Greek Orthodox church
Stakeholder	Being the adoptive parent of a hearing-impaired child
Legal identity	Recognized membership in a First Nation
Shared disease experience	Being a "breast cancer survivor"

Source: Derived from Davis (2000).

(NIH 2002a; NRC 1997). This potential interrelationship of community and individual consent highlights ethical issues that remain unresolved in the international research community—namely, whether individuals should be enrolled in a protocol if the community opposes the research, that is, whether a community veto should override an individual's decision to participate (Clayton 2002; NRC 1997). Community consent advocates note that individuals may always refuse participation even when the community has consented, and advise that when community consent is refused, individuals should not be approached for participation (Weijer and Emanuel 2000). Others criticize this latter point, noting that some community leaders may "systematically disenfranchise" some members of the group and infringe on their autonomy by attempting to deny their right to participate in research (Davis 2000). Some recommend that instead of seeking community consent, the individual informed consent process include discussion of risks and benefits to, and perhaps the objections of, the community; individuals can then weigh these issues in their decision about participation (Davis 2000; NBAC 1999; NRC 1997).

Dissemination of research results: privacy, pedigrees, and public understanding

Two sets of considerations present particular ethical concerns about dissemination of results of genetic research. First, as discussed earlier, genetic information has implications for families and for communities. Implications for families, however, are especially acute when pedigrees are published (Powers 1993). On the basis of information presented on the "family tree" itself (e.g., age, sex, age of disease onset, and relationship to other family members) and in the text of the publication (e.g., location of recruitment to the study, description of the condition and its symptoms), it may be possible to infer the identity of both families represented by, and individuals represented on, a published pedigree. The likelihood of inferential identification may vary in accordance with the condition studied. The consequences of such identification may vary in accordance with the condition, its treatability, the economic and social circumstances of those identified (e.g., their employment and insurance status, and what is already known about their or their family's condition, whether they live in a small town or large urban setting), and what incidental information is revealed on the pedigree (e.g., previously unacknowledged pregnancies or misattributed paternity). Access to a pedigree may result in an individual learning unwanted information about his own level of risk, as well as allowing others access to that information. In the absence of a more complete understanding of the ingredients of such risk analysis, however, the conclusions drawn may be inaccurate and lead to undue anxiety or a false sense of security, and ill-informed decision-making.

Because of these risks, many argue for the need to obtain informed consent to the publication of pedigrees (Botkin *et al.* 1998; Powers 1993). In light of the familial nature of genetic information and the possibility of group harms, however, such consent by one or even all family members in a study does not protect the privacy—the inaccessibility to identification—of nonparticipating family members (or nonconsenting study subjects). Omission of nonconsenting subjects from the pedigree is a mandatory and minimal response if one proceeds with publication; however, an incomplete pedigree may be misleading both scientifically and socially (i.e., leading to erroneous identifications and different sequelae, like false labeling). Undermining the study's scientific validity, and thus reducing its merit alters the risk:benefit calculation essential not only to justify publication of the results, but also to warrant investigators' conduct of the study and subjects' enrollment in it. Altering or falsifying data on the pedigree (e.g., changing birth order) or in the text (e.g., altering the study location) in an attempt to preserve anonymity is proscribed by the International Committee of Medical Journal Editors' guidelines for protecting privacy in publication (1995), although studies show that these guidelines fail to govern current practice (Bennett 2000; Botkin *et al.* 1998).

Investigators are asked to consider whether publication of a pedigree is necessary and whether a pedigree that is masked (e.g., by omitting all ages or sex of those represented) is sufficiently informative to warrant its potential misinformation risks. Any alteration or omission of information should be disclosed in the publication, as should the fact that consent to publication was obtained (Bennett 2000; International Committee 1995). In deciding whether to publish a pedigree, researchers should consider that rare conditions increase the risk of unwanted identification, and that greater harms may result from unwanted identification with respect to some conditions (e.g., psychiatric conditions), and some incidental information (e.g., reproductive history). In cases where the expected social benefit from the scientific knowledge shared through pedigree publication is so great that publication without explicit consent is considered, the likelihood of unwanted identification and subsequent negative sequelae must be sufficiently low to warrant a determination that publication presents only minimal risk, that is, "a very remote risk to privacy" (Powers 1993: 10).

Finally, concerns about unwanted identification and the difficulty of avoiding it without compromising the scientific value of publication should prompt consideration of alternate methods of sharing research results and making them available to scientists to evaluate and attempt replication (Powers 1993). Among these alternatives is the possibility of investigators publishing studies without inclusion of pedigrees and other details that may be necessary to enable replication, but agreeing to make such information available to other researchers who agree to take similar steps to protect the identity and privacy of subjects. This proposal demands careful consideration, as potential problems include the difficulty of determining who qualifies for access to the original investigators' pedigree data, and the diffusion of responsibility for failures of protective measures that result in unwanted identification.

The second set of considerations relevant to dissemination of results is less subject to regulation; it concerns the public's understanding of science and of genetic information in particular. Public understanding is an active, constructive faculty, not a mere state of lacking expert knowledge (Durant *et al.* 1996). At the same time, dissemination of research to the public often fuels what scientists would term public *mis*understanding. Media reports of "the discovery of the gene for X" result in simplistic views of gene–environment interaction, fatalistic beliefs, and risks of stigmatization. In addition, oversimplified public understanding of pharmacogenetics and gene therapy research has been fueled by efforts to garner public support for both enterprises. Pharmacogenetics' promise of individually tailored treatments summons images of physicians someday being able to select from a vast array of treatments the one specifically designed for a patient's genome, rather than a vision of orphaned populations of those who are nonresponsive to standard therapies suitable for the (profitable) majority. Gene therapy is described in terms of the precise surgical extraction and replacement of faulty segments of DNA. In terms of military analogies, the public views gene therapy as the sniper therapy, while the current reality might better be described in terms of well-working DNA groundtroops integrating alongside uncorrected genes and overwhelming the effect of faulty DNA in virtue of their sheer numbers. Scientists must take care to communicate accurately and strive to create realistic expectations of their research in both the general public and enrolled subjects.

Research on genetic testing: from analytical validity to clinical utility

Which ethical issues attach to research on genetic testing depend on (a) whether the test is under development, or is already validated, but being introduced into a particular population or clinical setting, and thus on (b) the goals of the study. A study to develop a test may seek to determine its analytic validity (i.e., its sensitivity, specificity, and predictive value with respect to genotype) or its clinical validity (i.e., those factors with respect to phenotype). Assessment of clinical utility (benefits and risks of testing and subsequent interventions) may be the goal of research on an already validated test (Khoury *et al.* 2000). Finally, the ethical issues depend in part on (c) the aim of the specific test being studied, just as they would were the test being employed in a clinical setting. Genetic tests may be developed for use in particular populations (e.g., newborn screening for galactosemia), or they may be diagnostic tests to confirm or exclude a suspected genetic disorder either in a fetus at risk for a condition, or in a symptomatic individual. Risk assessment tests—including, or sometimes also called, predictive or presymptomatic tests—are used in asymptomatic individuals to assess the probability that they will develop a particular condition, for example, HD (where a negative result excludes the diagnosis), or breast cancer (where testing may yield a lifetime risk greater than or roughly equal to that of the general population). The choice of population in which to demonstrate the effectiveness of a test or the feasibility of a screening program is ethically important. Many would argue that the choice of African Americans as the population for the implementation of one of the first population-based genetic screening programs was ethically problematic and exacerbated mistrust of the medicoscientific establishment by people of color (Andrews 1997; Bradby 1996; King 1998). Care must be taken to ensure that benefits and burdens of research participation are shared fairly by all members of society, especially when specific populations are to be targeted for testing. Care must also be taken to identify research questions and to design protocols for genetic testing research that minimize group harms, perhaps by employing community consultation, as discussed earlier.

Whether conducting research to develop a genetic test or to introduce a validated test into a population or clinical practice, assessment of what those receiving the test (or their parents) understand about the test and how they use test results, as well as the psychosocial sequelae of testing, will be of scientific interest, and will influence both the elements of informed consent and the nature of the ethical concerns that arise. If, for example, a particular newborn screening test were widely misunderstood and gave rise to substantial anxiety among parents, those outcomes would constitute an ethical concern, as well as a problem of clinical-scientific merit. Here the research ethics issues resemble those arising in the context of clinical trials, health services research, and research on psychosocial factors and health-related beliefs and behaviors. Research that involves giving the results of genetic tests to subjects raises all of the issues that clinical (or population-based) genetic testing does. In particular, the issues of informed consent and the need for genetic counseling are substantially the same. Protocols developed in the research context of HD testing, and later adapted for clinical testing, serve as a model for the incorporation of privacy and psychosocial safeguards, and genetic counseling into research on genetic testing (Harper 1993), although HD is distinguished by being an uncommon and as yet untreatable condition associated with substantial anxiety and stigma.

Research protocols that involve genetic testing without disclosure of test results to individuals, as when a test is under development, raise ethical issues similar to those described earlier, particularly concerns associated with nondisclosure of interim research results. If subjects forgo information or other interventions to which they would otherwise be entitled outside of the research context, special ethical concerns arise. A study to determine whether clinical outcomes may be improved by early risk assessment or diagnosis through genetic testing, for example, might involve withholding test results from an identified control group (Fost and Farrell 1989). Such research protocols must establish that asking subjects to forgo such putative benefits is justified, and the informed consent process must clearly explain the potential harms of doing so. Indeed if a standard of care has emerged, asking subjects to forgo that standard of care for the sake of answering a research question, no matter how great its social value, constitutes one of the most controversial research ethics questions of the late twentieth century (London 2000; Love and Fost 1997).

Gene transfer research: a special sort of clinical trial?

In the forthcoming revised *IRB Guidebook*, an entire chapter is to be devoted to gene transfer research. Such dedicated attention to issues that can only be sketched here seems justified for multiple reasons. First, despite arguments that somatic cell gene therapy should be viewed as "a natural and logical *extension* of current techniques for treating disease," and not as a qualitatively different type of intervention (Walters and Palmer 1997), the sociocultural significance of altering DNA complicates, and perhaps obscures, ethical analysis. Second, gene transfer research is subject to special regulatory oversight—specifically, joint oversight by the Food and Drug Administration (FDA) and the Recombinant DNA Advisory Committee (RAC) of the NIH—as well as the usual human subjects protections afforded under the Common Rule and through the oversight of the OHRP. This additional oversight is justified, in part, because few members of local IRBs have expertise in the science of gene transfer. A third consideration, though not unique to this context, may warrant protracted attention to the ethics of gene transfer research: the increasing role of commercial interests exacerbates the appearance, if not the reality, of conflicts of interest. Finally, gene transfer research raises all of the trial design issues and human subjects protection concerns presented by any clinical study.

Moreover, any discussion of ethical concerns must address the ethical missteps associated with the well-publicized death of gene therapy research subject Jesse Gelsinger in 1999. As former chair of the RAC LeRoy Walters said of gene therapy research at the time of Gelsinger's death, "until now, we have been able to say, 'Well it hasn't helped many people, but at least it hasn't hurt people'. That has changed." Indeed, Gelsinger's death dramatically underscored that "gene therapy research" is a confusing appellation. (Confusion was heightened in 1993 when, apparently under political pressure, the director of the NIH sparked controversy by granting a "compassionate use" exemption from established review procedures for the use of an experimental vaccine, created by gene transfer techniques, in a last-ditch attempt to trigger the immune system of a dying cancer patient (Thompson 1993).) Gene therapy research should not be confused with treatment, nor is it so-called therapeutic research. The ornithine transcarbamylase (OTC) deficiency trial that resulted in Gelsinger's death, for example, was a phase 1 trial whose goal was to test the safety, or maximally safe dose, of the transgenic vector; no individual therapeutic benefit was contemplated. The term "gene transfer research" is thus preferable.

The goal of gene transfer is to treat or prevent disease in individual patients by administering DNA rather than a drug. This is to be accomplished by correcting or enhancing the function of a mutated gene by supplying a normal copy of the gene, by directly correcting the mutated gene, or by introducing genetic material that regulates the expression of genes. To deliver the genetic material into the target cells, a variety of vectors, usually disabled viruses, have been used. In most cases the delivery of DNA must be conducted *in vivo* because removal of the target cells from the patient for *in vitro* administration of DNA is usually not practicable. Only somatic, not germline, cells may be targeted under current federal guidelines because of ethical and safety concerns about germline intervention (NIH 2002b).

Germline gene transfer

A variety of arguments are made against the pursuit of germline gene transfer. One consequence-oriented line of argument expresses concern about the possibility of unintended negative effects, tends to assume that such effects will be irreversible, and concludes, therefore, that these negative effects will be visited on successive generations of offspring. Rights-oriented lines of argument are often simultaneously invoked. One posits that future generations have a right to inherit a genome not subjected to human (or "artificial") intervention. Another suggests that research interventions targeting the germline subject future generations to research participation without their consent. Other arguments against pursuing germline gene transfer include its relatively limited applicability, given the (at least current) greater safety of other technologies like preimplantation genetic diagnosis; its anticipated relatively high cost, and thus the likelihood that only the well-off will afford its eventual benefit; its possible combination with phenotypic enhancement, and the perpetuation of such enhancement through generations; and its association with the destruction of embryos and totipotent embryonic cells, and attendant ethical concerns.

Arguments based on concern about unintended consequences must be evaluated in light of current scientific developments and standards of risk-taking commensurate with such standards in other contexts. Sociocultural commitments—including those reflected in the rights-oriented arguments—sometimes complicate the analysis to augur for a greater degree of risk aversion in this context than in other arenas that affect future generations (e.g., environmental interventions or wealth distribution policies). Arguments resting on the alleged distinction between the natural and unnatural are problematic, especially when applied to human genomes, because the genomes of living individuals and their offspring have always been affected by human interventions more and less directly, and usually quite inadvertently, for example, as medical and public health measures have allowed people to live and reproduce who otherwise would not, and as exposure to drugs and radiation have directly altered genes, including those in germ cells. A traditional distinction between therapy and enhancement is notoriously difficult to maintain (Juengst 1997, 1998; Resnik 2000), especially when it is noted that enhancement at the cellular level may restore "normal" phenotypic function (Torres 1997), or that some phenotypic enhancements may be justified on grounds of health, justice, or both (Buchanan *et al.* 2000; Rawls 1971: 107–08; Silvers 2002). That future offspring cannot consent to the research that results in changes to their genomes is true; no unborn individual consents to the conditions of his creation, nor do children consent to the interventions—standard or experimental—consented to by their guardians for their presumed benefit. (Nevertheless, complex ethical and metaphysical arguments—focused on welfare and on personal identity—may have relevance for assessment of gene transfer research that would affect embryos, fetuses, and perhaps as yet unconceived future generations (Wasserman 2002).) Avoidance of negative consequences, protection of rights, and provision of the circumstances of well-being for future generations require sound ethical decision-making about germline gene transfer, but articulation of these considerations does not itself constitute decisive arguments against it.

Concern that the well-off will be the primary beneficiaries of developments in the genetic revolution is justifiably raised about all genetic innovation, and perhaps most acutely about gene transfer research. Nevertheless, germline correction of genetic mutations associated with disease and disability, once effected, would be one putative benefit that is transmittable, without additional cost, through generations of both rich and poor alike. Given other social inequalities, for example in access to health care, it might be argued that the poor may benefit even more than the well-off from an absence of genetically increased risk of ill health (Resnik 1994).

Indeed, a variety of constituencies can reasonably raise arguments in support of eventually permitting germline gene transfer. Prospective parents may seek to spare their progeny from the results of deleterious genetic mutations, from being carriers of such mutations and having to make decisions about transmitting them, and from having to undergo somatic gene transfer themselves. The public and those concerned with the public's health may argue that it is best to prevent "once and for all" the effects of, and transmission of, disease-related genetic mutations, rather than having to intervene generation after generation. This line of reasoning is similar to the desirability of "wiping out" a severe contagious disease, rather than having to innoculate or treat each successive generation for it. Finally, there may be some conditions that must be prevented so early in the development of the human organism to avoid irreversible damage to the individual that the only way to prevent the damage is to intervene at such an early developmental stage that all cells, including germ cells, would be modified (Walters and Palmer 1997: 80–81).

Somatic cell gene transfer: trial design, regulatory oversight, and human subjects protections

Design

At present, however, gene transfer research is limited to somatic cells. Three basic questions of research design arise—namely, the identification of (1) an appropriate condition for study (i.e., for potential treatment by gene transfer), (2) an appropriate means of delivering the genetic material, and (3) an appropriate study population. In general, gene transfer research has centered on very serious or life-threatening conditions for which there is no good treatment. Introduction of the risks of gene transfer for less serious conditions, or where other reasonable alternatives exist, cannot be justified at the early—indeed phase 1—stage of gene transfer research. Another criterion for selection of a condition for study has been the relative, at least theoretical, ease of its treatment by gene transfer. Random integration of genetic material into the genome of target cells is easier to achieve than precise gene replacement or gene repair; therefore, conditions that have been ideal for early studies are those for which gene expression can be achieved relatively easily and for which the integration and activation of a small amount of "correct" genetic material would have a therapeutic effect. Thus, in contrast to conditions associated with complex gene regulation (e.g., hemoglobinopathies), diseases in which a single enzyme is missing have been ideal early candidates for gene transfer studies (e.g., OTC deficiency or adenosine deaminase deficiency). Other candidate conditions and treatment strategies for study have included cancers and attempts to introduce drug-sensitive genes into tumor cells and drug-resistant genes into noncancerous cells, or attempts to introduce "correct" copies of genes into cells in relevant tissues affected by recessive conditions (e.g., lung tissues in the case of cystic fibrosis).

Identification of both appropriate vectors and appropriate target tissues are trial design issues with ethical implications because of the relevance of such issues for the study's risk:benefit ratio, or in early studies with no prospect of benefit to subjects, the level of risk presented by the intervention. Genetic material has generally been introduced—first, *ex vivo*, and in later trials, *in vivo*—by vectors, often altered retroviruses that penetrate cells and integrate into a host genome with relative ease.

While less practicable *ex vivo* interventions present little risk of inadvertent germline gene transfer, *in vivo* interventions present a (presumably) small risk of inadvertent germline gene transfer (High 2003; King 2003; NIH 2002b).

Though not unique to the ethics of gene transfer research, identification of an appropriate study population is a critical question. Like all phase 1 research not suitable for enrollment of healthy volunteers, early gene transfer research enrolled human subjects with the condition under study who had no other good therapeutic alternatives. Moreover, limiting enrollment to seriously ill patients who were not sexually active or fertile eliminated the risk of inadvertent germline transfer. Such inadvertent transfer would occur through spread of vectors, and the genetic material they carry, to gonadal tissue, where such transgenic material could be passed on to offspring through subjects' subsequent reproductive activity.

Oversight and regulation

In addition to being subject to the usual regulatory and oversight provisions, including those governing research with human subjects, (federally funded) gene transfer protocols are reviewed by the RAC, which was created in 1974. In its early days, the RAC functioned as a sort of model national research ethics committee. It mandated creation of local Institutional Biohazard (or Biosafety) Committees at all institutions involved in (federally funded) recombinant DNA studies, and it conducted its business in open public meetings. This unusual measure was a response to public concern about the inadvertent release of recombinant DNA or new pathogenic organisms into the environment. As gene transfer research evolved from laboratory studies and animal models to clinical research, concern shifted from basic safety issues to human subjects protections. In 1983 the RAC formed an interdisciplinary Working Group on Human Gene Therapy and took on review of human gene transfer research protocols, alongside review by the FDA, which asserted its regulatory authority over gene transfer clinical trials in 1984 (Federal Register 1984) and again in 1993 (Federal Register 1993). The Working Group developed an extensive set of questions, "Points to Consider," that investigators seeking to conduct gene transfer trials must address (NIH 2002b).

In the early days of gene transfer studies in humans, the RAC imposed on investigators very stringent reporting requirements for adverse events. The rationale was that gene transfer technology was so new that it would be difficult for investigators to determine whether an adverse event was directly attributable to the gene transfer intervention. Therefore, the RAC required immediate reporting of all adverse events. In contrast, in keeping with its practice of treating gene transfer studies like trials of other biological drugs, the FDA required immediate reporting only of adverse events directly resulting from the study intervention and annual reporting of all other adverse events. As gene transfer research evolved further and various cancers and human immunodeficiency virus (HIV)/acquired immunodeficiency syndrome (AIDS) emerged as conditions of interest, cancer and AIDS activists joined researchers and members of the biotechnology industry in supporting gene transfer research and advocating for more streamlined processes for approving protocols.

The RAC's role became more advisory than regulatory. While some were concerned that a reduction in the RAC's authority would lead to a reduction in public account-ability surrounding gene transfer research, others advocated for relying on the FDA to provide the lion's share of federal regulatory oversight of gene transfer research.

Either reduction of regulatory oversight or confusion about regulatory authority and investigators' reporting responsibilities, or both, may have contributed to the 1999 death of Jesse Gelsinger. Consideration of both the circumstances leading to Gelsinger's death and the results of its investigation illustrates the interconnection of the regulatory, ethical, and trial design issues attending gene transfer research.

Lessons from the death of Jesse Gelsinger

At least in retrospect, it is possible to read accounts of the OTC deficiency study and Gelsinger's death as revealing regulatory failures, conflicting interests, and errors of judgment in addressing each of the three basic trial design issues sketched above. Nevertheless, the study also illustrates very traditional concerns about human subjects protections, including appropriate balancing of risks and benefits and the adequacy of informed consent.

OTC deficiency, caused by a missing or defective gene on the X chromosome, occurs in two forms: a very severe form typically affecting newborn males and a milder form that typically presents later. The missing gene results in the body's producing too little OTC, a liver enzyme that removes ammonia from the blood. The onset of the severe type occurs after affected children ingest protein. The first symptom is lethargy, followed by coma and often seizures. If the body's escalating ammonia level is not reversed, death soon results. Without liver transplantation, the majority of children with severe OTC deficiency suffer brain damage and die. The later-onset, milder form of the condition can be controlled by severely restrict-ing protein consumption and taking nutritional supplements. Gelsinger's OTC deficiency was diagnosed at age 2; he is a "mosaic" for the condition—that is, a small proportion of his cells produce the enzyme—and thus he suffers from the milder form of OTC deficiency.

OTC deficiency is in many ways a classic condition for studying gene transfer as a treatment. The basic rationale is that by supplying correct copies of missing or defec-tive gene, the body could be induced to produce adequate amounts of OTC. There are two forms of the disease that create two distinct study populations: newborns, who are incapable of giving informed consent to study participation themselves, but who generally have no good therapeutic alternative given the scarcity of livers for transplantation; and older children (capable of assenting to research participation) and adults (who might be able to give informed consent themselves), but who have a therapeutic alternative that is life preserving even if it impairs quality of life because of the strictness of the regimen. (Unaffected carriers constitute another possible study population. Indeed a large number of mothers of affected offspring volunteered, but the study was ultimately deemed too risky to enroll asymptomatic volunteers.)

The OTC deficiency study employed adenovirus as the gene transfer vector. Questions surrounded the method of introducing the vector into the body, as adenovirus had not been injected directly into the bloodstream before. While the RAC advised peripheral intravenous administration to reduce the likelihood of toxicity to subjects' liver tissue, the FDA requested infusion of the vector directly to the liver via the hepatic artery, in part, to minimize the risk of its dissemination to gonadal tissue (King 2003). Thus, it appears that choices of study design at least sometimes involve a trade-off between risks to subjects of somatic cell gene transfer research and the risk of inadvertent germline gene transfer (with attendant risks to the subjects' future offspring). So long as fertile, relatively healthy subjects are enrolled in gene transfer studies, concern to avoid inadvertent germline transfer is a consideration.

In the OTC deficiency study, severely ill newborns could have been chosen as the study population. Given the early stage, goal, and design of the study, those newborns would likely have died before having a chance to reproduce. The vector was to be administered only once, at least to initial trial participants, in gradually escalating doses for each group of 3 subjects, up to the total of 18 subjects. Instead of newborns, patients with the later-onset, milder form of OTC deficiency were chosen as the pool of potential subjects. The reason was, in part, because the consulting bioethicist raised concerns about the ability of parents of severely ill newborns to give voluntary informed consent to their children's trial participation. Although this rationale was supported by parents of such newborns and accepted by the RAC, at least in hindsight, this choice of study population seems misguided. It was unclear that parents of OTC deficient newborns would have had more difficulty giving valid informed consent than parents of children suffering from childhood cancers, who are allowed to consent to their children's study participation despite a trial's risks and no prospect of individual benefit. Moreover, to the extent that choice of study population, coupled with concern about inadvertent germline transfer by fertile subjects, led to the choice of a higher risk method of vector introduction, the rejection of newborns as subjects was misguided. In the OTC deficiency study, these choices led to the enrollment, in a phase 1 trial, of subjects for whom another therapeutic option existed, rather than the enrollment of subjects who had a very poor prognosis and no therapeutic options (unless transplantation was likely). Although it seems clear that Jesse Gelsinger (and his father) understood that he would derive no direct benefit from study participation, it is not clear that he (or his father) fully appreciated the risks it presented.

A final issue about enrollment criteria became salient in the case of Gelsinger's enrollment and infusion. In any clinical trial, enrollment inclusion and exclusion criteria are devised to ensure the scientific merit of the study and to protect research subjects. After Gelsinger's death, investigation of the application of the protocol's exclusion criteria suggested that while Gelsinger's ammonia levels were acceptable at the time of his enrollment, they were elevated above the stop level specified in the protocol at the time that the gene transfer vector was administered. This breach of protocol—or failure to interpret the protocol to afford maximal protection to subjects—was egregious. Upon review, such departure from the protocol was deemed especially suspicious because Gelsinger was the final subject to be tested and a variety of pressures to complete the trial could have been at play. That one of the investigators held the founding ownership interest in the biotechnology company that would benefit from success of the study gave rise to at least the appearance of a conflict of interest. The investigator, however, denied being influenced by financial interests and stated that he had taken pains to remain at arms length from the trial in human subjects (Smith and Byers 2002).

The appearance, and perhaps reality, of conflicting interests is not unique to either the OTC deficiency study or to gene transfer research. While the OTC deficiency study was NIH sponsored, a substantial number of gene transfer protocols have corporate sponsorship (Smith and Byers 2002), investigators often have financial interests in small biotechnology companies associated with gene transfer trials, and universities are increasingly encouraging technology transfer activities on the part of their faculty. However, such university–corporate partnerships, entrepreneurial activities on the part of university investigators, and the role of large and small corporations on clinical research are certainly not restricted to gene transfer research. Large-scale corporate-sponsored pharmaceutical trials enroll vastly larger numbers of subjects.

Controversy surrounds the question of whether potential conflicts of interest were adequately disclosed in the informed consent process in the OTC deficiency trial. Even more serious failures of disclosure did, however, impugn the validity of Gelsinger's informed consent. Investigation following his death revealed that previous adverse events, side effects of the investigational intervention, were not disclosed. At least two, perhaps four, of the previously infused subjects had suffered severe adverse effects, including significant liver stress. According to FDA regulations, these events should have been reported to the FDA and the study itself halted, but these requirements were not fulfilled. Moreover, it appears that investigators deleted information to be disclosed in the IRB-approved informed consent form to omit discussion of primate deaths in a previous, related study that had employed a stronger version of the adenovirus. Thus, although Gelsinger had an accurate understanding of the altruistic nature of his participation, he did not have relevant information regarding the attendant risks. Subsequent news reports quoted his father saying that he and his son viewed the study as "low risk" (Nelson and Weiss 1999; Stolberg 1999).

The investigation that followed Gelsinger's death, which investigators did promptly report to the FDA and NIH, revealed that nearly 700 adverse events from previous gene transfer studies had not been reported (Smith and Byers 2002). Some previous subjects had died, but whether their deaths were attributable to the gene transfer intervention is unknown. Whether Gelsinger's death was "the first gene transfer death" or not, in January 2000, the FDA suspended the OTC deficiency study, as well as other ongoing gene transfer trials. Discussion has ensued regarding the restructuring of regulatory oversight of gene transfer research. Nevertheless in mid-2000, the RAC accepted a plan that decreased its regulatory oversight and reduced redundancy of review by the RAC and Food and Drug Administration (FDA). At the same time, Congress initiated inquiries into the regulation of gene transfer research and commentators advocated for "helpful redundancy" and "public oversight." Specifically, commentators advocated for the adaptation of oversight mechanisms employed in multicenter phase 3 studies to the gene transfer context, with the creation of a combined statistical coordinating center and data safety monitoring board (either one centralized board or several, each focused on monitoring use of a particular vector or research on a particular condition) (Walters 2000). What is perhaps most striking about Gelsinger's death, however, is that the ethical concerns it illuminated are not unique to gene transfer research. Inadequate informed consent, regulatory failures, the possibility of conflicting interests, and ethical dimensions of trial design issues resolved in ways seen in retrospect to be ill advised—all are issues found in other research contexts.

Conclusion

It becomes evident that the ethics of the field of genetic research substantially overlaps with ethical issues in other research arenas. Distinct, perhaps, is the fact that with the exception of gene transfer research, genetic research is a "high tech" field of basic and applied science that presents primarily psychosocial risks. That risks arise for families and groups, not just individuals, is also distinctive. Also of ethical relevance is the special significance—cultural, ethical, religious, and social—that many people attach to genetic information and the biological material used to generate that information. For these reasons, the concerns that are associated with research on conditions—for example, on substance abuse, mental health, cancer, or even normal development— are intensified when the focus turns genetic. Rather than succumbing to such genetic exceptionalism or, on the other hand, failing to take seriously the public's perceptions and concerns, researchers and regulators would be well advised to treat genetic and nongenetic research as mutually informing realms of ethical inquiry as they attempt to balance interests and protect human subjects. Lessons from the ethical conduct of genetic research may have as far-reaching implications for research generally as genetic information does for generations.

Bibliography

American College of Medical Genetics: Storage of Genetic Materials Committee (1995) "Statement on Storage and Use of Genetic Materials," *American Journal of Human Genetics*, 57: 1499–500.

American Society of Human Genetics (2000) "Should Family Members about Whom You Collect Only Medical History Information for Your Research Be Considered 'Human Subjects'?," Online available: http://genetics.faseb.org/genetics/ashg/pubs/policy/pol-38.htm (accessed January 28, 2005).

——(1996) "Statement on Informed Consent for Genetic Research," *American Journal of Human Genetics*, 59: 471–74.

Andrews, L. (1997) "Past as Prologue: Sobering Thoughts on Genetic Enthusiasm," *Seton Hall Law Review*, 27: 893–918.

Appelbaum, P., Roth, L., and Lidz, C. (1982) "The Therapeutic Misconception: Informed Consent in Psychiatric Research," *International Journal of Law and Psychiatry*, 5: 319–29.

Bennett, R. (2000) "Pedigree Parables," *Clinical Genetics*, 58: 241–49.

Beskow, L.M., Botkin, J.R., Daly, M., Juengst, E.T., Lehmann, L.S., Merz, J.F., Pentz, R., Press, N.A., Ross, L.F., Sugarman, J., Susswein, L.R., Terry, S.F., Austin, M.A., and Burke, W. (2004) "Ethical Issues in Identifying and Recruiting Participants for Familial Genetic Research," *American Journal of Medical Genetics*, 130A(4): 424–31.

Botkin, J.R. (2001) "Protecting the Privacy of Family Members in Survey and Pedigree Research," *Journal of the American Medical Association*, 285: 207–11.

Botkin, J.R., McMahon, W.M., Smith, K.R., and Nash, J.E. (1998) "Privacy and Confidentiality in the Publication of Pedigrees," *Journal of the American Medical Association*, 279: 1808–12.

Bradby, H. (1996) "Genetics and Racism," in T. Marteau and M. Richards (eds) *The Troubled Helix: Social and Psychological Implications of the New Human Genetics* (pp. 295–316). Cambridge: Cambridge University Press.

Buchanan, A. (1998) "Testing and Telling: Implications for Genetic Privacy, Family Disclosure and the Law," *Journal of Health Care Law and Policy*, 1: 391–420.

Buchanan, A., Brock, D.W., Daniels, N., and Wikler, D. (2000) *From Chance to Choice: Genetics and Justice*, New York: Cambridge University Press.

Clayton, E. (2002) "The Complex Relationship of Genetics, Groups, and Health: What it Means for Public Health," *Journal of Law, Medicine, & Ethics*, 30: 290–97.

Clayton, E., Steinberg, K.K., Khoury, M.J., Thomson, E., Andrews, L., Kahn, M.J., Kopelman, L.M., and Weiss, J.O. (1995) "Consensus Statement: Informed Consent for Genetic Research on Stored Tissue Samples," *Journal of the American Medical Association*, 274: 1786–92.

Clinical Laboratory Improvement Amendments: 1988, 42 CFR 494.3(b)(2) Common Rule. 45 CFR 46.

Davis, D. (2000) "Groups, Communities, and Contested Identities in Genetic Research," *Hastings Center Report*, 30: 38–45.

Durant, J., Hansen, A., and Bauer, M. (1996) "Public Understanding of the New Genetics," in T. Marteau and M. Richards (eds) *The Troubled Helix: Social and Psychological Implications of the New Human Genetics* (pp. 235–48). New York: Cambridge University Press.

49 Fed. Reg. 50878 (December 31, 1984). Statement of Policy for Regulating Biotechnology Products.

58 Fed. Reg. 53248 (October 14, 1993) Application of Current Statutory Authorities to Human Somatic Cell Therapy Products and Gene Therapy Products.

Forrow, L., Arnold, R.M., and Parker, L.S. (1993) "Preventive Ethics: Expanding the Horizons of Clinical Ethics," *Journal of Clinical Ethics*, 4: 287–94.

Fost, N. and Farrell, P.M. (1989) "A Prospective Randomized Trial of Early Diagnosis and Treatment of Cystic Fibrosis: A Unique Ethical Dilemma," *Clinical Research*, 37: 495–500.

Foster, M. and Freeman, W.L. (1998) "Naming Names in Human Genetic Variation Research," *Genome Research*, 8: 755–57.

Foster, M., Eisenbraun, A.J., and Carter, T.H. (1997/1998) "Genetic Screening of Targeted Subpopulations: The Role of Communal Discourse in Evaluating Sociocultural Implications," *Genetic Testing*, 1: 269–74.

Foster, M.W., Bernsten, D., and Carter, T.H. (1998) "A Model Agreement for Genetic Research in Socially Identifiable Populations," *American Journal of Human Genetics*, 63: 696–702.

Harper, P. (1993) "Clinical Consequences of Isolating the Gene for Huntington's Disease," *British Medical Journal*, 307: 397–98.

High, K.A. (2003) "The Risks of Germline Gene Transfer," *Hastings Center Report*, 33(2): 3.

International Committee of Medical Journal Editors (1995) "Protection of Patients' Rights to Privacy," *British Medical Journal*, 311: 1272.

Juengst, E.T. (1998) "What Does 'Enhancement' Mean?," in E. Parens (ed.) *Enhancing Human Capacities: Conceptual Complexities and Ethical Implications* (pp. 29–47). Washington, DC: Georgetown University Press.

——(1997) "Can Enhancement be Distinguished from Prevention in Genetic Medicine?," *The Journal of Medicine and Philosophy*, 22(2): 125–42.

Khoury, M.J., Burke, W., and Thomson, E.J. (2000) "Genetics and Public Health: A Framework for the Integration of Human Genetics into Public Health Practice," in M.J. Khoury, W. Burke, and E.J. Thomson (eds) *Genetics and Public Health in the 21st Century* (pp. 3–24). New York: Oxford University Press.

King, N.M.P. (2003) "Accident Desire: Inadvertent Germline Effects in Clinical Research," *Hastings Center Report*, 33(2): 23–30.

King, P.A. (1998) "Race, Justice, and Research," in J.P. Kahn, A.C. Mastroianni, and J. Sugarman (eds) *Beyond Consent: Seeking Justice in Research* (pp. 88–110). New York: Oxford University Press.

London, A.J. (2000) "The Ambiguity and the Exigency: Clarifying 'Standard of Care' Arguments in International Research," *Journal of Medicine and Philosophy*, 25: 379–97.

Love, R.R. and Fost, N.C. (1997) "Ethical and Regulatory Challenges in a Randomized Control Trial of Adjuvant Treatment for Breast Cancer in Vietnam," *Journal of Investigative Medicine*, 45(8): 423–31.

Merz, J.F. (1996) "Is Genetics Research 'Minimal Risk'?," *Institutional Review Board*, 18(6): 7–8.

Mitchell, G. and Happe, K. (2001) "Informed Consent after The Human Genome Project," *Rhetoric and Public Affairs*, 4: 375–406.

National Bioethics Advisory Commission (NBAC) (1999) *Research Involving Human Biological Materials: Ethical Issues and Policy Guidance: Volume I*. Online available: www.georgetown. edu/research/nrcbl/nbac/hbm.pdf (accessed January 11, 2003).

National Institutes of Health (NIH) (2002a) "Bioethics Resources on the Web: Genetics: Points to Consider When Planning a Genetic Study that Involves Members of Named Populations," Online available: http://www.nih.gov/sigs/bioethics/named_populations.html (accessed December 9, 2003).

—— (2002b) *NIH Guidelines for Research Involving Recombinant DNA Molecules: Points to Consider in the Design and Submission of Protocols for the Transfer of Recombinant DNA Molecules into One or More Human Research Participants*, Appendix M. Online available: http://www4.od.nih.gov/ oba/rac/guidelines_02/Appendix_M.htm (accessed July 22, 2005).

National Research Council (NRC): Committee on Human Genome Diversity (1997) "Human Rights and Human Genetic-Variation Research," in *Evaluating Human Genetic Diversity* (pp. 55–68). Washington, DC: National Academy Press.

Nelson, D. and Weiss, R. (1999) "Family's Debate Mirrored Scientists' on Gene Therapy Risk," *The Washington Post*, September 30, A.07.

Office for Human Research Protection (OHRP) (2005) *Institutional Review Board Guidebook*, Washington, DC: Government Printing Office. Online available http://www.hhs.gov/ohrp/ irb/irb_guidebook.htm (accessed July 22, 2005).

—— (2004) *Guidance on Research Involving Coded Private Information of Biological Specimens*. Online available: http://www.hhs.gov/ohrp/humansubjects/guidance/cdebiol.pdf (accessed July 22, 2005).

Office for Protection from Research Risks (OPRR) (1993) *Protecting Human Research Subjects: Institutional Review Board Guidebook* (pp. 5:42–5:63). Washington, DC: National Institutes of Health.

Parker, L.S. (2002) "Ethical Issues in Bipolar Disorders Pedigree Research: Privacy Concerns, Informed Consent, and Grounds for Waiver," *Bipolar Disorders*, 4: 1–16.

—— (1994) "Bioethics for Human Geneticists: Models for Reasoning and Methods for Teaching," *American Journal of Human Genetics*, 54: 137–47.

Parker, L.S. and Lidz, C.W. (1994) "Familial Coercion to Participate in Genetic Family Studies: Is there Cause for IRB Intervention?," *Institutional Review Board*, 16(1–2): 6–12.

Pate v. Threlkel (358–60)661 So.2d, 278, 20 Fla. L. Weekly S35 (1995).

Powers, M. (1993) "Publication-Related Risks to Privacy: Ethical Implications of Pedigree Studies," *Institutional Review Board*, 15(4): 7–11.

Rawls, J. (1971) *A Theory of Justice*, Cambridge, MA: Belknap Press/Harvard University Press.

Reilly, P. (1998) "Rethinking Risks to Human Subjects in Genetic Research," *American Journal of Human Genetics*, 63(3): 682–85.

Resnick, D.B. (2000) "The Moral Significance of the Therapy—Enhancement Distinction in Human Genetics," *Cambridge Quarterly of Healthcare Ethics*, 9(3): 365–77.

——(1994) "Debunking the Slippery Slope Argument against Human Germ-Line Gene Therapy," *The Journal of Medicine and Philosophy*, 19(1): 23–40.

Safer v. Pack (361–68) 291 N.J.Super.619, 677 A.2d 1188 (1996).

Silvers, A. (2002) "Meliorism at the Millennium: Positive Molecular Eugenics and the Promise of Progress without Excess," in L.S. Parker and R.A. Ankeny (eds) *Mutating Concepts, Evolving Disciplines: Genetics, Medicine, and Society* (pp. 215–34). The Netherlands: Kluwer Academic Publishers.

Smith, L. and Byers, J.F. (2002) "Gene Therapy in the Post-Gelsinger Era," *JONA's Healthcare Law. Ethics, and Regulation*, 4(4): 104–10.

Stolberg, S.G. (1999) "The Biotech Death," *New York Times Magazine*, November 28, 136–50.

Thompson, L. (1993) "Should Dying Patients Receive Untested Genetic Methods?," *Science*, 259: 452.

Torres, J.M. (1997) "On the Limits of Enhancement in Human Gene Transfer: Drawing the Line," *The Journal of Medicine and Philosophy*, 22(1): 43–53.

Walters, L. (2000) "The Oversight of Human Gene Transfer Research," *Kennedy Institute of Ethics Journal*, 10(2): 171–74.

Walters, L. and Palmer, J.G. (1997) *The Ethics of Human Gene Therapy*, New York: Oxford University Press.

Wasserman, D. (2002) "Personal Identity and the Moral Appraisal of Prenatal Therapy," in L.S. Parker and R.A. Ankeny (eds) *Mutating Concepts, Evolving Disciplines: Genetics, Medicine, and Society* (pp. 235–64). The Netherlands: Kluwer Academic Publishers.

Weber, L. and Bissell, M.G. (2002) "Case Studies in Ethics: Socially Sensitive Research," *Clinical Leadership and Management Review*, 16: 244–45.

Weijer, C. (2000) "Benefit-Sharing and Other Protections for Communities in Genetic Research," *Clinical Genetics*, 58: 367–68.

——(1999) "Protecting Communities in Research: Philosophical and Pragmatic Challenges," *Cambridge Quarterly of Healthcare Ethics*, 8: 501–13.

Weijer, C. and Emanuel, E.J. (2000) "Protecting Communities in Biomedical Research," *Science*, 289: 1142–44.

Weijer, C., Goldsand, G., and Emanuel, E.J. (1999) "Protecting Communities in Research: Current Guidelines and Limits of Extrapolation," *Nature Genetics*, 23: 275–80.

Woodward, B. (1999) "Challenges to Human Subjects Protections in US Medical Research," *Journal of the American Medical Association*, 282: 1947–52.

4 Embryonic stem cell research and human therapeutic cloning

Maintaining the ethical tension between respect and research

Gerard Magill

The longstanding social contract that exists between society and science is increasingly under scrutiny and in jeopardy as we encounter the ever-changing landscape of biotechnology today. Recent breakthroughs in embryonic stem cell research and human therapeutic cloning have raised the stakes even higher, both for science and policy discourse. And at the heart of the many debates about these neuralgic issues is the ethical tension between promoting respect for human dignity and promoting research for medical therapies. However we may want to characterize the so-called social contract between society and science, there is little doubt that society's investment in, and support of, basic and applied research is closely connected with society's responsibility for, and commitment to, respect for human dignity. And however we may describe the longstanding tension between what can be identified metaphorically as the "tectonic plates" of respect and research, there can be little doubt about the deep rumblings being caused by their clashing in the debate on embryonic stem cell research and human therapeutic cloning. This debate has become perhaps the main fault line for exposing the seismic tension between the "tectonic plates" of human respect and medical research in today's technologically driven society.

This chapter seeks to maintain the ethical tension between respect and research in the debate on embryonic stem cell research and human therapeutic cloning. It would be a reach too far to seek a resolution of this tension, not only because it would be too difficult to attain, but above all because it would be mistaken to do so. After all, a profound respect for human dignity over many centuries has inspired many scientific discoveries and inventions. In turn, the abundance of insight and accomplishment over centuries in basic and applied research has enhanced the flourishing of society by celebrating human dignity. Recognizing the constructive nature of this tension between respect and research does not mean there have not been many problems or negative results, the experiments in the Holocaust being the most obvious. This chapter seeks to foster the constructive nature of the tension between respect and research in the debate on embryonic stem cell research and human therapeutic cloning as a crucial foundation for policy discourse today.

The analysis begins with a brief case study to highlight the tension between respect and research in stem cell research. Then, the analysis connects the emergence of embryonic stem cell research with the related policy and ethics debates and concludes with an ethical review of the connection between embryonic stem cell research and human therapeutic cloning. The analysis seeks to calibrate the seismic tension between the metaphorical "tectonic plates" of respect and research as a volatile but unavoidable foundation for constructing reliable policy structures in today's complex society.

Preimplantation genetic diagnosis and stem cell donation

Ethics discussion of preimplantation genetic diagnosis (PGD) has increased over recent years to consider the legitimacy of applying this new technology for many different purposes, such as screening embryos for susceptibility to cancer, for Alzheimer's disease or diabetes, and very controversially for human leukocyte antigen (HLA) matching for tissue donation to an existing child.[1]

In the late 1990s, the first case to combine PGD with stem cell transplant was that of Molly and Adam Nash. Molly Nash had a rare genetic disorder (Fanconi anemia) preventing her body from making bone marrow. This condition can kill at a very young age. Molly was 6 years old. A bone marrow transplant from a matching sibling can offer an 85 percent rate of success for treating this disease, but Molly did not have a sibling. Hence, her parents opted to have another baby hoping to use the placenta and cord blood for a stem cell transplant. This involved three separate interventions and technologies. They used *in vitro* fertilization (IVF) for assisted reproduction at the Colorado Center for Reproductive Medicine in Denver, PGD at the Reproductive Genetics Institute in Chicago, and stem cell transplantation at the University of Minnesota. These interventions ensured that the future baby did not have the same disease as Molly and that there would be a good match for the transplant. On August 29, 2000, baby Adam was born. After three weeks and further screening, his sister received transfusion of stem cells from his umbilical cord and placenta: bone marrow recovery occurred within a week or so.[2] Both Adam and Molly flourished, and years later Molly has a normal immune system. This intervention was the first recorded experiment that merged the three technologies of IVF, PGD, and HLA matching for the stem cell transplant.

However, these interventions were not without ethical controversy. A widely recognized question clearly concerns the ethical status of the human embryos created to select an appropriate match for treating a sibling, especially with regard to treating them as persons with rights or as property for medical research.[3] In this case, fifteen human embryos at eight-cell stage were created via IVF; some were discarded and baby Adam was born. But there are many other questions that ethics discourse needs to address. A recent ethics study of these issues recommended the following practical guidelines. First, research protections need to be applied when creating a donor child by adopting appropriate research protocols, specifically adopting the category of greater than minimal risk but offering the direct benefit to the research subject (the donor child). Second, the sibling's health condition should be life threatening or seriously disabling, establishing that significant benefits to the affected sibling may outweigh the potential burdens on the mother and the donor child. Third, IVF and PGD procedures should be preceded by psychological evaluation of the parents to assess their ability to rear the donor child without subsequent exploitation. Fourth, risks faced by the donor child should not be increased in order to benefit the recipient sibling, thereby honoring research regulations to permit risk when it is justified by anticipated benefits to the subjects involved. Fifth, prior to subsequent invasive harvesting procedures from the donor child, there should be independent psychological evaluation of the parents and the donor child when age appropriate. Sixth, even before the donor child is competent to make decisions, risks or burdens to the donor child should be limited carefully based on justifying risk (which, after birth, are most likely to be psychosocial) by anticipated benefit to the donor child. Seventh, there should be only a limited number of testing and harvesting procedures, for example, when considering the need for bone marrow harvest(s) if the initial stem cell harvest and transplant fails. Eighth, the donor child should have an independent physician who is committed solely to protecting and advancing the child's best interests. Finally, any harvesting procedure should require both parental permission and ethics review (Wolf *et al.* 2003).

These practical guidelines provide a good example of the constructive tension between promoting respect for human dignity and promoting research for medical therapies. On the one hand, the guidelines seek to safeguard the future interests of the donor child; on the other hand, the guidelines promote a research focus with appropriate protocols. This constructive tension between respect and research urges us to establish a sound framework for evaluating what risks, burdens, and limits may be appropriate, to clarify what consent is necessary, and to address the conflicts that parents face as they decide for their donor child while trying to save the older sibling.

The Nash case illustrates today's high hopes for stem cell therapies, even though there are many related ethical concerns about the tension between promoting respect for human dignity and promoting research for medical therapies. Not least, there are important concerns with patient safety and efficacy, such as in a failed stem cell experiment on patients with Parkinson's disease that involved sham surgery (Freed *et al.* 2001).[4] However, new expectations for stem cell therapies have been increased in an extraordinary manner by breakthroughs in embryonic stem cell research. And just as concerns with creating and destroying human embryos in the IVF–PGD process in the Nash case elicit extensive ethical scrutiny, the debate on the moral status of the embryo has dominated the debate on embryonic stem cell research that typically entails both the creation and destruction of the human embryo. However, like the Nash case, it could be mistaken reductivism to narrow this complex ethical debate to that single issue.

The emergence of embryonic stem cell research

Breakthroughs in 1998 in embryonic stem cell research and embryonic germ cell research fueled the ethical debate about using these cells for basic research and cell-based treatments and therapies (Shamblot *et al.* 1998; Thomson *et al.* 1998). Mouse embryonic stem cells were derived much earlier, in 1981 (Evans and Kaufman 1981; Martin 1981). In 1998, scientists at the University of Wisconsin-Madison led by Professor James Thomson (using spare embryos from infertility laboratories), in collaboration with Geron Corporation (Menlo Park, CA), and scientists at The John Hopkins University led by John Gearhart (using aborted fetal tissue), announced separate successful experiments in isolating and culturing embryonic human stem cells using somatic cell nuclear transfer. This process replicated the technology pioneered by Ian Wilmut at the Roslin Institute in Edinburgh, Scotland to clone the famous ewe Dolly in 1997 (Wilmut and Schnieke 1997).[5]

The hopes for stem cell research are to revolutionize both drug development and the testing process used by pharmaceuticals and biotechnology companies. The 1998 breakthrough in embryonic stem cell research was immediately accompanied by an expansive literature.[6] Faced with such promise, it is imperative to distinguish realistic expectations from the specter of false hopes that can be such a disservice to the sick and disabled (Dresser 2003a).

In 2002, the National Academy of Sciences published a report urging further attention to the potential importance of stem cell research for regenerative medicine (NRC/IOM 2001/2002). Two years later, in early 2004, the President's Council on Bioethics published a report on stem cell research, including a survey of progress in embryonic stem cell research. The purpose of the President's Council includes several goals that can be construed reasonably as akin to the tension being discussed in this essay, the tension between respect for human dignity and research for medical therapies. These goals include pursuing inquiry into the human and moral significance of developments that occur in biomedical and behavioral science and technology; addressing ethical and policy questions related to these developments; providing a forum for national discussion of bioethical issues; and facilitating greater understanding of bioethical issues, including international collaboration. President George Bush originally appointed this Council to address many of the emerging issues in biotechnology. After producing a report on human cloning (2002), the Council turned to stem cell research (2004). However, politics were very much part of the process as became clear when, without any public reason, two Council members were not reappointed in spring 2004. This caused controversy about the Council's credibility and its diverse set of views and positions; one of the members who was not reappointed subsequently published a critique of the Council's work accusing it of misrepresenting research on human aging and stem cells.[7]

The Council began its report on stem cell research by a helpful explanation of the types of stem cells and why there is ethical debate about their use (President's Council on Bioethics 2004: 1–20).[8] Stem cells refer to multipotent cells that are relatively undifferentiated in the sense that they give rise to specialized cells of the body. A pluripotent cell can produce all the cell types of the developing organism; multipotent cells are more specialized but can produce multiple differentiated cell types. All stem cells are capable of self-renewal and are capable of producing differentiated descendent cell types. Embryonic stem cells are derived from the inner cell mass of the blastocyst after the zygote has divided to approximately 200 cells. The inner cell mass develops into the body of the embryo; the outer trophoblast cells develop into the placenta etc. to support the embryo's development. In contrast, embryonic germ cells are stem cells isolated from the gonadal ridge of a fetus (whereas fetal stem cells are derived from the organs and tissues as the fetus develops). These germ cells develop into sperm or egg cells, according to the sex of the fetus. These cells can be harvested from fetuses aged 5 to 9 weeks, donated after induced abortions. Currently, federally funded research on embryonic germ cells is permitted as governed by federal regulations. The development process moves from the original germ cells of the parents to fertilization, after which the zygote proceeds to the first cleavage and subsequent cell divisions. In the process of implantation, the blastocyst forms: its outer form develops into the trophoblast (which develops into the placenta and other supporting structures), and its inner form develops into the inner cell mass that develops into the embryo. As the inner cell mass develops, the primitive streak begins to appear, which has become a very important boundary in policy discussions about research on human embryos. Subsequently, neurulation is a developmental process that results in the beginning of the central nervous system, and organogenesis indicates the development of the basic structures for the emergence of major organ systems in the fourth to eighth week.[9]

Adult stem cells are more differentiated (hence the term "adult") than embryonic stem cells or embryonic germ cells. These nonembryonic cells can generate lineages of more specialized cells within the same broad type of tissue (muscle, etc.), but they are typically considered to be less versatile or flexible because of their differentiation. They are found in the tissue of fetuses, children, and adults. The use of adult stem cells in research raises few ethical concerns, other than the usual obligation to obtain consent and balance benefits with risk, etc. Finally, cord blood stem cells are a nonembryonic form. Hematopoietic stem cells and other progenitor cells can be isolated from the blood in the umbilical cord in the hope of developing subsequent stem cell treatments that are likely to circumvent rejection problems of other donors (President's Council on Bioethics 2004: 8–11).

From a scientific perspective, stem cells facilitate the study of cellular and developmental processes. From a medical perspective, stem cells provide a source of cells and tissues that can be transplanted for repair and regeneration. Pursuing these possibilities has led to an intense policy debate that sheds light on the underlying tension between promoting respect for human dignity and research for medical therapies.

The emergence of the policy debate on embryonic stem cell research

Understanding federal funding of research is crucial to grasping the policy debate on stem cell research (President's Council on Bioethics 2004: 21–51).[10] Current federal funding policy is best understood in the context of the history of the funding debate on embryo research.

In the wake of the abortion debate after *Roe v. Wade* (1973), the US Congress issued a temporary moratorium on federal funding for research using a living human fetus, unless seeking the survival of the fetus. Congress established a National Commission for the Protection of Human Subjects of Biomedical and Behavioral Research to offer guidelines for human fetal and embryo research for funding standards. When the Commission issued its report in 1975, the statutory moratorium was lifted.

The Commission called for a national Ethics Advisory Board within the Department of Health, Education, and Welfare (DHEW) to offer guidelines about federal funding of research on human embryos. The Ethics Advisory Board was established in 1975 and issued its report in 1979 (its charter ended in 1980 with no renewal or replacement) (DHEW 1979). Its report suggested that research on embryos was ethically defensible but controversial. The DHEW decided against providing federal funding for human embryo research. In 1993 Congress passed the NIH Revitalization Act in which it rescinded the need for research protocols to be approved by a then nonexistent Ethics Advisory Board. This made National Institutes of Health (NIH) funding of human embryo research possible.

In 1994 the NIH convened a Human Embryo Research Panel to propose guidelines for federal funding of such research. The Panel recommended federal funding of some human embryo research, including the creation of human embryos to use them for research (NIH 1994a,b). President Clinton did not accept the latter recommendation, but implemented the former using embryos left over from IVF procedures. But Congress intervened in 1995 before any NIH funding was approved for research on human embryos, with a prohibitive provision (the "Dickey Amendment").[11] The provision forbad the creation of human embryos for research purposes, banned research whereby human embryos could be destroyed, discarded, or knowingly subjected to risk of injury or death (greater than what is permitted for research on fetuses in utero), and the meaning of the term human embryo included organisms derived by fertilization, parthenogenesis, cloning, or other means from human gametes or human diploid cells.[12] It is important to emphasize that the law did not prohibit research using private funding. Hence, at the federal level, there is no support or prohibition of privately funded research that involves destroying human embryos. Although this law preceded the isolation of human embryonic stem cells in 1998 via privately funded research at the University of Wisconsin, Congress has reenacted the Dickey Amendment every year since 1995. Subsequently, a legal interpretation of the law argued that only research "in which" embryos were destroyed was forbidden, thereby permitting federally funded research on embryos that were destroyed previously by privately funded researchers. The subsequent policies of President Clinton and President Bush accepted this approach.

In response to public expectation, two reports were presented by the National Bioethics Advisory Commission (NBAC) and by the NIH. In 1999, the NBAC presented a lengthy report, *Ethical Issues in Human Stem Cell Research*, and in August 2000, the NIH published its revised guidelines on embryonic stem cell research with the support of President Clinton.[13] The NIH guidelines permitted the use of federally funded research to derive human pluripotent stem cells from fetal tissue (derived by agencies not supported by federal funding), provided there was informed consent of the donors and no financial inducement. The NIH guidelines sought to establish a distance between the derivation of embryonic stem cells (involving a process that destroys the embryo) and federally funded research on embryonic stem cells. In summer 2000, President Clinton's administration permitted federally funded embryonic stem cell research on embryos left over from reproduction IVF procedures, donated in accordance with standards of informed consent and free of financial inducements (though the guidelines were not implemented or funded because of the change in administration). A study published in 2003 indicates that approximately 400,000 embryos are stored in the United States, with 88.2 percent being targeted for patient use (Hoffman *et al.* 2003). This leaves a very small percentage for research, such as in embryonic stem cell technology.[14]

One year later, on August 9, 2001, President Bush announced his policy that would permit public funding of embryonic stem cell research, but in a more restrictive fashion than his predecessor (President's Council on Bioethics 2004: 183–87).[15] Prior to his announcement, the NIH presented a report to encourage policy and ethics debate (NIH 2001). President Bush approved federal funding for approximately sixty genetically diverse stem cell lines. These lines came from stem cells via the previous destruction of human embryos. He was determined to defend the principle that federal funds should not support the future destruction of human embryos in such research while maximizing the good that could be obtained from preexisting stem cell lines developed previously (even though the destruction of human embryos was involved). Yet, many consider this to be a distinction without any effective difference (e.g., Robertson 1999; Spike 2003). However, for advocates of human life, this distinction is a very important one to make if the constructive tension between respect for human dignity and research for medical therapies is to be maintained.

President Bush's policy statement claimed there were approximately sixty of these preexisting genetically diverse stem cell lines across the world that could receive federal funding for research. In September 2003, the NIH presented a list of the lines across the globe that were eligible for funding, but not necessarily available for use (President's Council on Bioethics 2004: 89–190). In fact, in fall 2003, substantively fewer lines were actually available for use. However, many consider the cell lines may be unsuitable for use in human trials and treatments, or that the lines do not have sufficient genetic diversity for research needs and therapies, thereby making this policy unsustainable.[16] The NIH established an online human embryonic stem cell registry to accept applications for federal grants and to list stem cell colonies approved for federally funded research.[17] Despite the policy of President Bush to restrict federal funding to develop new embryonic stem cell lines, private funding continues to facilitate their development elsewhere. Recent figures suggest there are approximately ten US companies pursuing embryonic stem cell research, spending in excess of $70 million of private funds for this research, in addition to federal NIH funding.[18] For example, in spring 2004, privately funded research at Harvard University derived multiple embryonic stem cell lines from human blastocysts. This research reports the derivation and characterization of seventeen new human embryonic stem cell lines. These new lines are in addition to the currently reported fifteen human embryonic cell lines that are publicly available (though reportedly difficult to obtain, difficult to maintain, and poorly characterized) and eligible for federally funded research (Phimister and Drazen 2004). Because the research involved the destruction of human embryos after the policy statement of President Bush in August 2001, these cell lines may not be used in research that is federally funded. The researchers obtained 286 frozen human embryos that had been produced via IVF for clinical purposes. Written consent and approval by a Harvard University Institutional Review Board were obtained. The research cultured the thawed embryos (at the cleavage stage of 6 to 12 cells each) to the blastocyst stage; 58 frozen and thawed blastocysts were reexpanded in culture (many of the embryos were of such poor quality that they did not further develop after thawing); the researchers then isolated 97 inner cell masses and derived 17 human embryonic stem cell lines (Cowan *et al.* 2004; Johannes and Regaldo 2004). There are scientific advantages and disadvantages to this accomplishment. On the one hand, these cell lines were cultivated in the presence of penicillin and streptomycin, whereas most embryonic stem cell lines available previously were intolerant of antibiotics. These cell lines are available for other scientists by using a "Material Transfer Agreement" for noncommercial research purposes and not using federal funds. On the other hand, these cell lines were grown on layers of mouse feeder cells, thereby raising the specter of interspecies transfer of viruses, though the Food and Drug Administration (FDA) has not yet forbidden the clinical use of such potential cell-based therapies (Gearhart 2004a).

The policy debate on embryonic stem cell research continues in the US Congress. A possible constraint upon embryonic stem cell research slipped into law in January 2004. The US Congress approved in its "Consolidated Appropriations Act, 2004" a prohibition of issuing patents (via the US Patent and Trade Office) on human organisms: "None of the funds appropriated or otherwise made available under this Act may be used to issue patents on claims directed to or encompassing a human organism" ("Consolidated Appropriations Act" 2004).[19] Opponents argue that the legislative language was unclear (e.g., no definition of human organism was included), and the measure was not debated on the floor, with no hearing in the House or the Senate. Representative David Weldon, the Florida Republican, added the law to the omnibus spending bill thereby forcing opponents to reject the measure in the highly unpalatable but only way possible, by voting against the entire spending bill. Representative Weldon provided assurances that his policy would not interfere with existing patents on stem cells and that the word "organism" does not include stem cells. Nonetheless, opponents fear that the bill could forbid patents on many human-derived biotechnology inventions and could be a backdoor legislative effort to stifle therapeutic cloning research. These opponents subsequently lobbied Congress to prevent the inclusion of this provision in the budget approval process.

The policy debate on embryonic stem cell research also continues to flare internationally, as is evident from the legal inconsistencies in Europe, and the political maneuvers at the United Nations.[20] In August 2001, France and Germany proposed a UN convention against human reproductive cloning, banning it in nations that ratified the convention. In February 2002, the United States joined the Vatican in seeking to expand the proposed convention to include both reproductive cloning and therapeutic cloning for research purposes. In fall 2003, at the Fifty-Eighth Session of the UN General Assembly, a two-year deferral of further debate prevailed by a vote of 80 in favor of deferral (including France, Germany, and the United Kingdom) to 79 votes against deferral (including the United States) with 15 abstentions. Despite this significant setback, Costa Rica introduced a resolution in December 2003 to ban all human cloning. A compromise was reached whereby Costa Rica agreed not to raise the resolution when the two-year deferral was reduced to one year, thereby scheduling an international convention on reproductive human cloning for a subsequent General Assembly. The debate was dominated by two opposing camps: Costa Rica, the United States, and the Vatican as the most prominent opponents of all kinds of human cloning; Belgium, France, Germany, and the United Kingdom as the most prominent proponents of banning only human reproductive cloning and permitting human therapeutic cloning. Also, the Organization of the Islamic Conference adopted a position indicating that early embryos and five-day-old blastocysts do not command protection as human subjects and are akin to other human cells that may be transplanted (Walters 2004).

In light of these policy debates, a patchwork legal framework emerged in the United States.[21] The existing legal framework includes bans on cloning with some exceptions for research, bans on embryo research, and laws addressing embryonic stem cell research, and there are several proposed bills on reproductive cloning, on therapeutic cloning, and on embryonic stem cell research (Andrews 2004).

The emergence of the policy debate on embryonic stem cell research suggests that, in our increasingly pluralistic and technological societies, viable policy options are constructed upon recognition of the underlying tension between respect for human dignity and research for medical therapies. Properly calibrating the metaphorical seismic tension between these "tectonic plates" of respect and research is indispensable for the construction of sufficiently flexible policies to withstand the inevitable "quakes" that ethics and cultural differences can create. And the ethics debate on embryonic stem cell research has become, metaphorically, perhaps the main fault line for exposing the seismic tension between the "tectonic plates" of respect and research.

The emergence of the ethics debate on embryonic stem cell research

The integration of ethics with science and public policy is crucial for the debate on embryonic stem cell research.[22] The developing ethical debate on embryonic stem cell research posits many claims and counterclaims, including a continuum of issues from the use of biased language in ethics, to empirical arguments in ethics, to the use of relevant ethical principles for decision-making (President's Council on Bioethics 2004: 53–108).[23] And the ethical tension between promoting respect for human life and promoting research for medical therapies is undoubtedly at the heart of this public discourse. Hence, there is an indispensable need to balance respect for human dignity with promising medical research on embryonic stem cells that may lead to new therapies and treatments for many diseases and debilities.

Some argue that the duty to relieve pain and suffering should be an overriding principle for biomedical science and research, outweighing concerns for frozen embryos that could be used in embryonic stem cell research. Others contend that defending moral principles does not entail responsibility for those who are suffering from diseases because possible treatments should not be developed by research that is forbidden (Callahan 2003). For example, many insist that the promise of research should never compromise respect for human life (Doerflinger 2002; Fitzgerald 2002; Green 2002a; Latham 2002; Orr 2002; Weissman 2002). Certainly, the ongoing debate about the moral status of the human embryo cannot be underestimated in this policy debate, not least because of its connection to underlying assumptions, as occurs, for example, in the support for donating spare embryos for research by the NRC/IOM for Reproductive Medicine (Ethics Committee of the American Society for Reproductive Medicine 2002).[24]

It is not surprising that much of the ethical debate about the legitimacy of embryonic stem cell research revolves around the perceived moral status of the embryo, though some argue that granting personal status to an embryo does not necessarily prevent killing it.[25] However, some regret such an association as an inappropriately framing of the debate in individualistic terms, seeking rather to expand the debate to engage larger related issues, such as social justice, commodification, and boundary issues related to human flourishing when we encounter merging human and non-human species in science research (Lauritzen 2004: 247–63).[26] It may be enticing to compare this disagreement about embryonic stem cell research with the longstanding debate on abortion. But it is unlikely that the abortion paradigm can help to resolve the debate about embryonic stem cell research. After all, in 1973 *Roe v. Wade* (410 US 113(1973)) was resolved by the US Supreme Court as a matter of the mother's right to privacy founded in the Fourteenth Amendment's view of personal liberty.[27] The right to the mother's privacy does not pertain in the debate on embryonic stem cells insofar as the embryos in question exist independently from the mother.

It seems more likely that the ethics debate on embryonic stem cell research might benefit from the earlier debate on fetal tissue research.[28] This debate goes back at least to the late 1970s. In 1978, IVF technology was pioneered by Robert Steptoe and Patrick Edwards with the birth of Louise Brown (DHEW 1979; Edwards and Steptoe 1978, 1980). And in 1979, the US Ethics Advisory Board indicated it was ethical to create research embryos to investigate safety issues with IVF technology. This debate flared as a result of the famous *Warnock Report* (1985a) and the approvals in Britain and Canada of creating and using research embryos, including the NIH, *Report of the Human Embryo Research Panel* (1994).[29] Like the debate on fetal tissue research, ethical debate on the status of the early embryo has been vibrant for a considerable time,[30] including influential perspectives in religious ethics.[31]

This debate on the status of the early embryo will continue to influence regulatory policies about embryonic stem cell research.[32] Rather than adopt a reductive stance that could compromise the constructive tension between respect and research, the debate on the status of the early embryo should foster discourse on other ethical concerns about embryonic stem cell research that are crucial to developing effective regulatory policies for our pluralistic societies. The President's Council on Bioethics considered other ethical challenges in its 2004 report, emphasizing the following areas:[33] further investigation into stem cells derivatives; further scrutiny of reproducible results using stem cell preparations and their derivatives; further understanding of human stem cells, including human adult stem cells (such as mesenchymal stem cells, multipotent adult progenitor cells, neural stem cells), human embryonic stem cells, and embryonic germ cells; further study of basic research using human stem cells; further analysis of human stem cells and the treatment of disease; and further inquiry about private sector activity.

The Council's report offered no recommendations, but drew the following preliminary conclusions: human stem cells can be reproducibly isolated from embryonic, fetal, and adult tissue sources; research using human stem cell preparations hold promise not only for increased understanding of the basic molecular process in cell differentiation and of the early stages of genetic disease, but also for future cell transplantation therapies for human diseases and disabilities; stem cell based therapies and treatments require both basic and applied research for a long time ahead; and transplant rejection problems remain a major obstacle for such therapies.

These many ethical concerns about embryonic stem cell research will continue to elicit dynamic debate, integrating science, ethics, and policy. Cumulatively, these issues and debates reflect the underlying tension between respect for human dignity and research for medical therapies. And the constructive tension between these "tectonic plates" of respect and research is indispensable for the construction of effective regulatory policies as viable structures for our pluralistic societies. Although it could be reductive to let any single issue trump the others in such policy formulations, it is increasingly likely that one topic will dwarf the others as we continue to integrate science, ethics, and policy in discussing embryonic stem cell research. The topic is that of human therapeutic cloning.[34]

The emergence of the ethics debate on human therapeutic cloning

Ethics discourse on human therapeutic cloning, whereby human embryos are created (and then destroyed) to harvest embryonic stem cells for research purposes, raises an extensive range of controversial issues. These issues range from contrasting therapeutic cloning with the use of surplus IVF embryos,[35] to connecting human cloning with germline gene therapy,[36] to commodification concerns,[37] to identity compromise,[38] to considering species related issues.[39] The policy and ethics debate will haunt legislators, especially in Europe and the United States, for many years to come.[40]

In June 1997, the NBAC published a report on human cloning arguing that, because safety concerns posed undue risk to potential offspring, there should be a federal ban against both reproductive and therapeutic cloning.[41] Congress did not act on this recommendation. Subsequently, NBAC published another report in September 1999, permitting the destruction of human embryos for medical research, limiting its recommendation to spare embryos only and not applying its analysis to therapeutic cloning.[42] A few months later, in June 2000, Liam Donaldson, Britain's chief medical officer, presented a report on stem cell research recommending therapeutic cloning in Britain to facilitate medical research on human embryonic stem cells (UK Department of Health 2000).[43] Parliament accepted the nine recommendations, introducing legislation to amend the "Human Fertilisation and Embryology Act" (1990) in statutory legislation.[44] This previous 1990 Act permitted targeted research on embryonic tissues obtained via aborted fetuses or spare embryos from IVF techniques.[45]

In the United States, a dramatic breakthrough in human cloning occurred on November 25, 2001 when Advanced Cell Technology in Worcester, Massachusetts, announced that it had successfully cloned human embryos. The experiment was unsuccessful insofar as the researchers had been unable to develop and harvest embryonic stem cells (Cibelli *et al.* 2001, 2002).[46] Ethicist Ronald Green, then chair of the ethics advisory board for Advanced Cell Technology and director of the Ethics Institute at Dartmouth College, explained that most members of the ethics board did not consider the organism produced by therapeutic cloning as equivalent to any ordinary human embryo because it did not result from the normal egg/sperm fertilization process.[47]

As a result of the above developments in human cloning, a clear demarcation of opposing viewpoints emerged, especially on using therapeutic cloning to harvest embryonic stem cells for medical research versus seeking alternatives to human cloning.[48] The US Congress was under more pressure than ever to resolve the policy debate on embryonic stem cell research and human therapeutic cloning,[49] especially to ensure that ethics discourse influences science and research policy in this emerging field.[50]

In the wake of these developments, the President's Council on Bioethics published a report on human cloning in 2002.[51] The report on human cloning resulted after six months of discussion, research, and deliberation (starting in January 2002). The selection of human cloning for a Council report was in part based on safety concerns of cloning techniques, potential medical benefits from cloning research, and moral concerns about experimenting on human embryos. More deeply, the topic was selected because of concerns about the impact of the research imperative in biotechnology upon human freedom, equality, and dignity.

The Council considered several public policy options for the report, including professional self-regulation without federal legislative action, a ban on reproductive cloning with no endorsement or restriction of therapeutic cloning, a ban on reproductive cloning with regulation of therapeutic cloning, government regulation of both reproductive and therapeutic cloning, a ban of all human cloning, a ban on reproductive cloning with a moratorium on therapeutic cloning, a moratorium on all cloning (President's Council on Bioethics 2002: 195–223).

However, the Council could not reach unanimity and made several recommendations (President's Council on Bioethics 2002: 225–56). With a unanimous voice, the Council held that reproductive cloning to produce children is both unsafe and unethical and, therefore, should be banned by federal law.[52] It argued that reproductive cloning would violate the ethical principles of human research, especially in light of the pervasive safety issues surrounding cloning of other mammals. The Council could see no ethical way, now or in the future, to discover whether reproductive human cloning could become safe. Based upon the ethical principles of respecting human freedom, equality, and dignity, the Council identified five major categories of concern about reproductive cloning: concerns about the identity and individuality of cloned children; concerns about the meaning of manufacturing children (who could be perceived more as products than gifts), thereby commercializing or industrializing the process of human procreation; concerns about the prospect of a new eugenics, such as by genetically engineered enhancements; concerns about troubled family relations by transgressing the natural boundaries between generations; and concerns about the effects on society, such as changing the way society looks at children (President's Council on Bioethics 2002: 83–129).

Apart from this unanimous recommendation to ban reproductive cloning, the other recommendations from the Council had split votes. First, a majority of ten members recommended a ban on reproductive cloning combined with a four-year moratorium on therapeutic cloning that would apply to researchers regardless of federal research funds being used.[53] The majority group also recommended a federal review of human embryo research, PGD, and genetic modification of human embryos and human gametes to foster public consensus, and shape ethically sound policies. Second, a minority of seven members recommended a ban on reproductive cloning but with federal regulations supporting therapeutic cloning whereby cloned embryos could be used for biomedical research.[54] The minority group recognized that such research could generate crucial information about human embryological development and gene activity, potentially leading to treatments and even cures for many diseases and disabilities. However, the members also recognized the controversial nature of such research insofar as it entails the deliberate production, use, and destruction of cloned human embryos that technically could be implanted to produce cloned children (President's Council on Bioethics 2002: 131–94). A number of arguments on each side of the debate about therapeutic cloning were considered. The case in favor of therapeutic cloning is based, for the most part, upon the quest by medical practitioners and biomedical researchers to relieve human suffering. This perspective accords no special moral status to the early cloned embryo. The case against therapeutic cloning readily acknowledges the future possibility of therapies from this research. Nonetheless, this position considers it to be morally wrong to exploit and destroy developing human life.

In sum, there was unanimous opposition to reproductive cloning. In addition, the majority members of the Council recommended a four-year moratorium on therapeutic cloning, while the minority members of the Council sought to permit therapeutic cloning with strict federal regulations. In spring 2004, the ethics and policy stakes in the debate on therapeutic cloning were raised significantly when a team of scientists in South Korea announced a substantive breakthrough in their research on human therapeutic cloning.

In February 2004, the first successful human cloning to generate embryonic stem cells was accomplished by a team of researchers in South Korea (Hwang *et al.* 2004; Phimister and Drazen 2004). They reported the derivation of human embryonic stem cells from a human cloned blastocyst. The study showed the feasibility of generating human embryonic stem cells from a somatic cell isolated from a living person. As a result of this breakthrough there will be increasing pressure upon scientists, ethicists, and policy makers to ascertain whether human therapeutic cloning should be permitted to advance research in embryonic stem cell research. Once again, the status of the human embryo in the debate on human therapeutic cloning, as in the debate on embryonic stem cell research, encapsulates in an extraordinarily clear way the tension between respect for human dignity and research for medical therapies. It is unlikely that human reproductive cloning will cloud the debate on human therapeutic cloning, especially given the widespread opposition to reproductive human cloning discussed earlier. Undoubtedly, the policy and ethics debate will revolve around the tension between human respect and medical research that has been discussed in this chapter.

Conclusion

The debate on embryonic stem cell research and human therapeutic cloning has become perhaps the main fault line, metaphorically speaking, for exposing the seismic tension between the "tectonic plates" of promoting respect for human dignity and promoting research for medical therapies. This essay has argued to maintain the constructive nature of the ethical tension between human respect and medical research as a crucial foundation for constructing viable policies in our pluralistic societies.

The case of Molly and Adam Nash provides a timely example of this tension, not least because of the successful outcome of stem cell therapy. Much more controversially than such stem cell therapies, embryonic stem cell research raises many policy and ethical issues that also revolve around the fundamental tension between respect and research. Not surprisingly, the debate on the status of the early embryo encapsulates this tension in an extraordinarily clear way, with the potential to elicit extreme advocacy stances, either in the name of respect for human dignity or in the name of research for medical therapies. However, permitting such extreme stances on either side to trump the other is likely to compromise the constructive nature of this important tension between respect and research. There is an appealing alternative to any reductive stance that could compromise this important and fundamental tension. The alternative is to seek appropriate connections between the debate on the status of the early embryo and other crucial issues about embryonic stem cell research that reflect and enhance the underlying tension between respect and research. Yet, despite the reluctance to let one advocacy stance trump other positions in this debate about embryonic stem cell research, it is likely that human therapeutic cloning could dwarf many other valid topics.

The importance of maintaining the ethical tension between respect and research is evident in the cited reports from the President's Council on Bioethics. That is, the Council's goals can be construed reasonably as being akin to fostering this tension between respect for human dignity and research for medical therapies, as discussed in this essay. Maintaining this ethical tension between respect and research can provide a foundation for effective regulatory policies in our pluralistic societies. In other words, viable policy options can be built upon recognition of the constructive tension between promoting respect for human dignity and promoting research for medical therapies. This essay has argued that calibrating the metaphorical seismic tension between these "tectonic plates" of respect and research is indispensable for the construction of sufficiently flexible policies to withstand the inevitable "quakes" that ethics and cultural differences can create. Like a proverbial earthquake, this underlying tension between the "tectonic plates" of respect and research could cause extensive damage in society if the tension goes unnoticed. The hope of this essay is to notice the tension and to recognize its constructive nature in the sense of identifying a major fault line upon which viable policy structures can be constructed. But let there be warning: seismic tensions should be approached warily.

Notes

1 For example, Robertson (2003a,b). For a reply, see Ashcroft (2003). See also Towner and Loewy (2002).
2 See Clancy (2001), Pennings *et al.* (2002), Robertson *et al.* (2002), Savulescu (2002), Verlinsky *et al.* (2001).
3 See Lauritzen (2001a), Meyer and Nelson (2001).
4 The experiment involved forty Parkinson's patients, aged 34–75. *Substantia nigra* cells from four aborted fetuses (6–10 weeks) were either transplanted into their brains *or* the patient received sham surgery. No overall benefit resulted, but significant side effects such as serious writhing occurred in some younger patients. For a report on genomic screening of Parkinson disease, see Scott *et al.* (2001). For critical ethical reviews, see Dekkers and Boer (2001), Macklin (1999). Also see Friedrich (2002).
5 Wilmut originally opposed using the technique of cloning for human medicine. See Wilmut (1998).
6 For a scientific introduction to stem cell biology in general and embryonic stem cells in particular, see Marshak *et al.* (2001), especially Chapters 1 and 10. For a representative sample of the early literature following the scientific breakthrough in 1998, see Abkowitz (2002), Chapman *et al.* (1999), Keller and Snodgrass (1999), Meyer (2000), "Symposium: Human Primordial Stem Cells" (1999), Weissman (2002).
7 The two members of the Council were Elizabeth H. Blackburn and William F. May. The critique was published on a website (Blackburn and Rowley 2004). A protest letter to President Bush was signed by 174 bioethicists and posted on the website of the *American Journal of Bioethics* ("Open Letter to President Bush," 2004).
8 For a general analysis of the importance of stem cell research for social policy and ethics, see Harris (2003). Harris argues for adopting a "principle of waste avoidance" to justify embryonic stem cell research. Also see Harris (1992, 1998).
9 For a scientific summary, see President's Council on Bioethics (2004: 157–81).
10 See Berkowitz (2004).
11 The amendment originally was attached to the Departments of Labor, Health and Human Services, and Education, and Related Agencies Appropriations Act in 1995. The "Dickey Amendment" was named after its author, then Representative Jay Dickey of Arkansas.
12 Parthenogenesis occurs via egg cells whose chromosomes are both from the mother but still begin normal embryonic development. Scientists at Advanced Cell Technology and at the Institute for Reproductive Medicine and Genetic Testing in Los Angeles are working on deriving stem cells through parthenogenesis. See Kaebnick (2001).
13 See also Fletcher (2000). A related, earlier document is DHEW (1979). For some scholarly commentary, see Kirk (2000), Marwick (1999), Mikes (2001), Rosso (1999), Wildes (1999).
14 Only 2.8 percent (approximately 3,000) of embryos from IVF clinics are donated for research (Hoffman *et al.* 2003).
15 For the text of the television address by President George Bush, see "Address on Federal Funding of Embryonic Stem Cell Research" (2001). Also see Alta Charo (2001a), Hanna (2001), Meilander (2001).
16 See, for example, Capron (2002), Dawson *et al.* (2003), Faden *et al.* (2003).
17 To access the registry, see http://stemcells.nih.gov/registry/index.asp

18   The name and number of derived lines can be found in President's Council of Bioethics (2004: 42–47), citing Lysaught and Hazlehurst (2003).

19   See Wilkie (2004).

20   For a review of developments in Europe, see Matthiessen (2001), Romeo–Casabona (2002).

21   See, for example, Shapiro (2003).

22   See, for example, Holland *et al.* (2001).

23   Also see Cheshire (2004), Harris (2002), Heinemann and Honnefelder (2002), Holm (2002, 2003), Lauritzen (2004), Solbakk (2003).

24   The view of respecting the embryo while not according it full personal rights was included in the report of NBAC (1999: ii and 2). Also see Green (2001b), London (2002), McCartney (2002), McGee (2002), Mahowald and Mahowald (2002), Meyer and Nelson (2001), Steinberg (2002), Strong (1997), Sullivan (2003).

25   See, for example, Outka (2002), Savulescu (2002).

26   Also see, for example, Faden *et al.* (2003), Holland (2001), Lauritzen (2001b), Resnik (2002).

27   See Noonan (1973), Tribe (1988: 1341–42). The Court's decision created a virtually unconditioned right of abortion especially when read together with the Court's decision on the same day in *Doe v. Bolton* (410 US 179(1973)). For a more detailed analysis of this debate, see Rainey and Magill (1996), especially the introduction.

28   For a historical review of fetal tissue research and its connection with stem cell research, see Cassell (2001).

29   See also Human Fertilisation and Embryology Authority (Great Britain) (1998), NIH (1994b), Royal Commission on New Reproductive Technologies (1993), Warnock (1985b).

30   For example, Cahill (1993, 1997), Cataldo (2001), Ford (1988, 2001, 2002), Johnson (1995), McCormick (1991), McGee and Caplan (1999), Porter (1995), Shannon (1997), Shannon and Wolter (1990), Steinbock (1992), Suarez (1990), Tauer (1997).

31   For example, see Cioffi (2002), Doerflinger (2001), Parker (2001).

32   For example, see Alta Charo (2001b), Campbell (2001), Juengst and Fossel (2000), Keenan (2001), Lauritzen (2001b), Ryan (2001), Shannon (2002), Steinbok (2001).

33   The appendices of the report contain several essays that were invited, including Gearhart (2004b), Itescu (2004a,b), Jaunisch (2004), Ludwig and Thomson (2004), Prentice (2004), Verfaillie (2004).

34   See Magill (2002, 2004).

35   See, for example, Hansen (2002).

36   See Willgoos (2001).

37   See Coors (2002).

38   See Agar (2002).

39   See Baylis (2002).

40   For example, Annas (2002), Annas *et al.* (2002), Evers (2002).

41   For a critique of this 1997 NBAC decision, see Green (2001b: 113–19).

42   For a critique of this 1999 NBAC decision, see Green (2001b: 158–63).

43   Also see a subsequent report confirming the Donaldson report, UK Department of Health (2002).

44   See *The Human Fertilisation and Embryology (Research Purposes) Regulations 2001*. Also see *The Human Reproductive Cloning Act* (2001) that was passed in response to a High Court judgment on November 15, 2001 that "embryos created by cell nuclear replacement were not governed by the Human Fertilisation and Embryology Act 1990." The passage of British legislation to ban reproductive cloning was intended to close a loophole in previous legislation that approved human therapeutic cloning. Also see Documentation Column (2002), Klotzko (2002), Sleator (2000).

45   See Committee on the Ethics of Gene Therapy (1992), Dziobon (1999), Gene Therapy Advisory Committee (1997).

46   The accomplishment elicited sturdy advocacy opposition; see Martino (2001).

47 For an earlier perspective on related research by a competing corporation, see Lebacqz, *et al.* (1999). For an earlier essay on human cloning research by several scholars including Ronald Green, see Lanza *et al.* (2000). Also see Green (2001a,b, 2002b).

48 For example Cohen (2001), Fitzgerald (2001), Hanson (2001), Kass and Wilson (1998), Lauritzen (2001b), Robertson (1999).

49 For insightful essays on public policy issues on cloning, see section three in Forsetr and Ramsey (2001), Lauritzen (2001b), including Tauer (2001), Moreno and London (2001), Stiltner (2001).

50 See Knowles (2000/2001).

51 Also see Childress (2003), Dresser (2003a,b).

52 For a philosophical analysis of the related arguments, see Häyry (2003).

53 The majority members were Rebecca Dresser, Francis Fukuyama, Robert George, Mary Ann Glendon, Alfonso Gómez-Lobo, William Hurlbut, Leon Kass, Charles Krauthammer, Paul McHugh, and Gilbert Meilander.

54 The minority members were Elizabeth Blackburn, Daniel Foster, Michael Gazzaniga, William May, Janet Rowley, Michael Sandel, and James Wilson.

Bibliography

Abkowitz, J.L. (2002) "Can Human Hematopoietic Stem Cells Become Skin, Gut, or Liver Cells?," *New England Journal of Medicine*, 346(10): 770–72.

"Address on Federal Funding of Embryonic Stem Cell Research," (2001) *Origins*, 31: 213–15.

Agar, N. (2002) "Cloning and Identity," *Journal of Medicine and Philosophy*, 28(1): 9–26.

Alta Charo, R. (2001a) "Bush's Stem Cell Compromise: A Few Mirrors?," *Hastings Center Report*, 31(6): 6–7.

——(2001b) "Every Cell is Sacred: Logical Consequences of the Argument from Potential in the Age of Cloning," in P. Lauritzen (ed.) *Cloning and the Future of Human Embryo Research* (pp. 82–91). New York: Oxford University Press.

Andrews, L.B. (2004) "Legislators as Lobbyists: Proposed State Regulation of Embryonic Stem Cell Research, Therapeutic Cloning and Reproductive Cloning," in *Monitoring Stem Cell Research: A Report of the President's Council on Bioethics*, Appendix E (pp. 199–224). Washington, DC: President's Council on Bioethics.

Annas, G.J. (2002) "Cloning and the US Congress," *New England Journal of Medicine*, 346(20): 1599–602.

Annas, G.J., Andrews, L.B., and Isasi, R.M. (2002) "Protecting the Endangered Human: Toward an International Treaty Prohibiting Cloning and Inheritable Alterations," *American Journal of Law & Medicine*, 28: 151–78.

Ashcroft, R. (2003) "Back to the Future," *Journal of Medical Ethics*, 29(4): 217–19.

Baylis, F. (2002) "Human Cloning: Three Mistakes and an Alternative," *Journal of Medicine and Philosophy*, 27(3): 319–37.

Berkowitz, P. (2004) "The Meaning of Federal Funding," in *Monitoring Stem Cell Research: A Report of the President's Council on Bioethics*, Appendix F (pp. 225–36). Washington, DC: President's Council on Bioethics.

Blackburn, E. and Rowley, J. (2004) "Reason as Our Guide," *PLOS Biology*, 2: 4. Online available: http://www.plosbiology.org (accessed October 11, 2004).

Cahill, L.S. (1997) "The Status of the Embryo and Policy Discourse," *Journal of Medicine and Philosophy*, 22: 407–14.

——(1993) "The Embryo and the Fetus: New Moral Contexts," *Theological Studies*, 54: 124–42.

Callahan, D. (2003) *What Price Better Health: The Hazards of the Research Imperative*, Los Angeles, CA: University of California Press.

Campbell, C.S. (2001) "Source or Resource? Human Embryo Research as an Ethical Issue," in P. Lauritzen (ed.) *Cloning and the Future of Human Embryo Research* (pp. 34–49). New York: Oxford University Press.

Capron, A. (2002) "Stem Cell Politics: The New Shape to the Road Ahead," *American Journal of Bioethics*, 2(1): 35–36.

Cassell, J.H. (2001) "Lengthening the Stem: Allowing Federally Funded Researchers to Derive Human Pluripotent Stem Cells from Embryos," *University of Michigan Journal of Law Reform*, 34: 547–72.

Cataldo, P. (2001) "Human Rights and the Human Embryo," *Ethics & Medics*, 26: 1–2.

Chapman, A.R., Frankel, M.S., and Garfinkle, M.S. (1999) *Stem Cell Research and Applications: Monitoring the Frontiers of Biomedical Research*, Washington, DC: American Association for the Advancement of Science and the Institute for Civil Society.

Cheshire, W.P. (2004) "Human Embryo Research and the Language of Moral Uncertainty," *The American Journal of Bioethics*, 4(1): 1–24.

Childress, J. (2003) "Human Cloning and Human Dignity: The Report of the President's Council on Bioethics," *Hastings Center Report*, 33(3): 15–18.

Cibelli, J.B., Kiessling, A., Cunniff, K., Richards, C., Lanza, R.P., and West, M.D. (2001) "Somatic Cell Nuclear Transfer in Humans: Pronuclear and Early Embryonic Development," *The Journal of Regenerative Medicine*, 2: 25–31.

Cibelli, J.B., Lanza, R.P., West, M.D., and Ezzell, C. (2002) "The First Human Cloned Embryo," *Scientific American*, 286(1): 44–51.

Cioffi, A. (2002) "Reproductive and Therapeutic Cloning," *Ethics & Medics*, 27(3): 1–3.

Clancy, F. (2001). "A Perfect Match," *Medical Bulletin* [Minnesota Medical Foundation], (Winter) 15–17.

Cohen, C.B. (2001) "Banning Human Cloning—Then What?," *Kennedy Institute of Ethics Journal*, 11: 205–09.

Committee on the Ethics of Gene Therapy (1992) *Report of the Committee on the Ethics of Gene Therapy: The Clothier Report*, London: Her Majesty's Stationary Office.

"Consolidated Appropriations Act, 2004," *HR* 2673, Sec. 634.

Coors, M.E. (2002) "Therapeutic Cloning: From Consequence to Contradiction," *Journal of Medicine and Philosophy*, 27(3): 297–317.

Cowan, C.A., Klimanskaya, I., McMahon, J., Atienza, J., Witmyer, J., Zucker, J.P., Wang, S., Morton, C.C., McMahon, A.P., Powers, D., and Melton, D.A. (2004) "Derivation of Embryonic Stem-Cell Lines from Human Blastocysts," *New England Journal of Medicine*, 350(13): 1353–56.

Dawson, L., Bateman-House, A.S., Mueller Agnew, D., Bok, H., Brock, D.W., Chakravarti, A., Greene, M., King, P.A., O'Brien, S.J., Sachs, D.H., Schill, K.E., Siegel, A., Solter, D., Suter, S.M., Verfaillie, C.M., Walters, L.B., Gearhart, J.D., and Faden, R.R. (2003) "Safety Issues in Cell-Based Intervention Trials," *Fertility and Sterility*, 80(5): 1077–85.

Dekkers, W. and Boer, G. (2001) "Sham Neurosurgery in Patients with Parkinson's Disease: Is it Morally Acceptable," *Journal of Medical Ethics*, 27: 151–56.

Department of Health, Education and Welfare (DHEW) (1979) *Report and Conclusions: Support of Research Involving Human In Vitro Fertilization and Embryo Transfer*, Washington, DC: Government Printing Office.

Documentation Column (2002) "The Status of the Embryo: The House of Lords Select Committee Report," *The Tablet* (March 9): 31–32.

Doe v. Bolton 410 US 179 (1973).

Doerflinger, R. (2002) "Ditching Religion and Reality," *American Journal of Bioethics*, 2(1): 31.

—— (2001) "The Policy and Politics of Embryonic Stem Cell Research," *The National Catholic Bioethics Quarterly*, 1(2): 135–43.

—— (1999) "The Ethics of Funding Embryonic Stem Cell Research: A Catholic Viewpoint," *Kennedy Institute of Ethics Journal*, 9: 137–50.

Dresser, R. (2003a) "Embryonic Stem Cells: Expanding the Analysis," *American Journal of Bioethics*, 2(1): 40–41.

—— (2003b) "Human Cloning and the FDA," *Hastings Center Report*, 33(3): 7–8.

Dziobon, S. (1999) "Germ-line Gene Therapy: Is the Existing UK Norm Ethically Valid?," in A.K. Thompson and R.F. Chadwick (eds) *Genetic Information: Acquisition, Access, and Control* (pp. 255–65). New York: Kluwer Academic/Plenum Publishers.

Edwards, R. and Steptoe, P. (1980) *A Matter of Life*, New York: William Morrow.

—— (1978) "Birth after Reimplantation of a Human Embryo," *Lancet*, 2: 336.

Ethics Committee of the American Society for Reproductive Medicine (2002) "Donating Spare Embryos for Embryonic Stem-Cell Research," *Fertility and Sterility*, 78(5): 957–60.

Evans, M.J. and Kaufman, M.H. (1981) "Establishment in Culture of Pluripotential Cells from Mouse Embryos," *Nature*, 292: 154–56.

Evers, K. (2002) "European Perspectives on Therapeutic Cloning," *New England Journal of Medicine*, 346(20): 1579–82.

Faden, R.R., Dawson, L., Bateman-House, A.S., Agnew, D.M., Bok, H., Brock, D.W., Chakravarti, A., Gao, X.J., Greene, M., Hansen, J.A., King, P.A., O'Brien, S.J., Sachs, D.H., Schill, K.E., Siegel, A., Solter, D., Suter, S.M., Verfaillie, C.M., Walters, L.B., and Gearhart, J.D. (2003) "Public Stem Cell Banks: Considerations of Justice in Stem Cell Research and Therapy," *Hastings Center Report*, 33(6): 13–27.

Fitzgerald, K. (2002) "Questions Concerning the Current Stem Cell Debate," *American Journal of Bioethics*, 2(1): 50–51.

—— (2001) "Cloning: Can It be Good for Us? An Overview of Cloning Technology and Its Moral Implications," *University of Toledo Law Review*, 32: 327–36.

Fletcher, J.C. (2000) "The National Bioethics Advisory Commission's Report on Stem Cell Research: A Review," *ASBH Exchange*, 3(1): 8–11.

Ford, N.M. (2002) *The Prenatal Person: Ethics from Contraception to Birth*, Oxford: Blackwell Publishers.

—— (2001) "The Human Embryo as a Person in Catholic Teaching," *The National Catholic Bioethics Quarterly*, 1(2): 155–60.

—— (1988) *When Did I Begin?*, New York: Cambridge University Press.

Forsetr, H. and Ramsey, E. (2001) "The Law Meets Reproductive Technology: The Prospect of Human Cloning," in P. Lauritzen (ed.) *Cloning and the Future of Human Embryo Research* (pp. 201–21). New York: Oxford University Press.

Freed, C.R., Greene, P.E., Breeze, R.E., Tsai, W.Y., DuMouchel, W., Kao, R., Dillon, S., Winfield, H., Culver, S., Trojanowski, J.Q., Eidelberg, D., and Fahn, S. (2001) "Transplantation of Embryonic Dopamine Neurons for Severe Parkinson's Disease," *New England Journal of Medicine*, 344: 710–19.

Friedrich, M.J. (2002) "Research Yields Clues to Improving Cell Therapy for Parkinson Disease," *Journal of American Medical Association*, 287(2): 175–76.

Gearhart, J. (2004a) "New Human Embryonic Stem Cell Lines—More is Better," *New England Journal of Medicine*, 350(13): 1275–76.

—— (2004b) "Human Embryonic Stem Cells: June 2001–July 2003. The Published Record," in *Monitoring Stem Cell Research: A Report of the President's Council on Bioethics*, Appendix H (pp. 273–77). Washington, DC: President's Council on Bioethics.

Gene Therapy Advisory Committee (1997) *Third Annual Report*, London: Health Departments of the UK.

Green, R. (2002a) "Determining Moral Status," *American Journal of Bioethics*, 2(1): 28–29.

——(2002b) "Benefiting from Evil: An Incipient Moral Problem in Human Stem Cell Research and Therapy," *Bioethics*, 16: 544–56.

——(2001a) "Much Ado about Mutton: An Ethical Review of the Cloning Controversy," in P. Lauritzen (ed.) *Cloning and the Future of Human Embryo Research* (pp. 114–31). New York: Oxford University Press.

——(2001b) *The Human Embryo Research Debates: Bioethics in the Vortex of Controversy*, New York: Oxford University Press.

Hanna, K.E. (2001) "Stem Cell Politics: Difficult Choices for the White House and Congress," *Hastings Center Report*, 31(4): 9.

Hansen, J.E.S. (2002) "Embryonic Stem Cell Production through Therapeutic Cloning has Fewer Ethical Problems than Stem Cell Harvest from Surplus IVF Embryos," *Journal of Medical Ethics*, 28: 86–88.

Hanson, M.J. (2001) "Cloning for Therapeutic Purposes: Ethical and Policy Considerations," *University of Toledo Law Review*, 32: 355–65.

Harris, J. (2003) "Stem Cells, Sex, and Procreation," *Cambridge Quarterly of Healthcare Ethics*, 12: 353–417.

——(2002) "The Ethical Use of Human Embryonic Stem Cells in Research and Therapy," in J. Burley and J. Harris (eds) *A Companion to Bioethics* (pp. 158–74). Oxford: Blackwell.

——(1998) *Clones, Genes, and Immortality*, New York: Oxford University Press.

——(1992) *Wonderwoman and Superman: The Ethics of Biotechnology*, New York: Oxford University Press.

Häyry, M. (2003) "Philosophical Arguments for and against Human Reproductive Cloning," *Bioethics*, 17(5–6): 447–59.

Heinemann, T. and Honnefelder, L. (2002) "Principles of Ethical Decision Making Regarding Embryonic Stem Cell Research," *Bioethics*, 16(6): 530–43.

Hoffman, D.I., Zellman, G.L., Fair, C.C., Mayer, J.F., Zeitz, J.G., Gibbons, W.E., and Turner, T.G., Jr (2003) "Cryopreserved Embryos in the United States and Their Availability for Research," *Fertility and Sterility*, 79: 1063–69.

Holland, S. (2001) "Contested Commodities at Both Ends of Life: Buying and Selling Gametes, Embryos, and Body Tissues," *Kennedy Institute of Ethics Journal*, 11(3): 266.

Holland, S., Lebacqz, K., and Zoloth, L. (eds) (2001) *The Human Embryonic Stem Cell Debate: Science, Ethics, and Public Policy*, Cambridge, MA: The MIT Press.

Holm, S. (2003) "The Ethical Case against Stem Cell Research," *Cambridge Quarterly of Healthcare Ethics*, 12: 372–83.

——(2002) "Going to the Roots of the Stem Cell Controversy," *Bioethics*, 16(6): 494–507.

Human Fertilisation and Embryology Act (1990) London: Her Majesty's Stationery Office.

Human Fertilisation and Embryology Authority (Great Britain) (1998) *Code of Practice*, 4th edn, London: Paxton House.

Human Fertilisation and Embryology (Research Purposes) Regulations 2001 (2001) London: Her Majesty's Stationery Office.

Human Reproductive Cloning Act (2001) London: Her Majesty's Stationery Office.

Hwang, W.S., Ryu, Y.J., Park, J.H., Park, E.S., Lee, E.G., Koo, J.M., Jeon, H.Y., Lee, B.C., Kang, S.K., Kim, S.J., Ahn, C., Hwang, J.H., Park, K.Y., Cibelli, J.B., and Moon, S.Y. (2004) "Evidence of a Pluripotent Human Embryonic Stem Cell Line Derived from a Cloned Blastocyst," *Science*, 303: 1669–74. March 12 (published online February 12). Online available: www.sciencexpress.org (accessed October 12, 2004).

Itescu, S. (2004a) "Stem Cells and Tissue Regeneration: Lessons from the Recipients of Solid Organ Transplantation," in *Monitoring Stem Cell Research: A Report of the President's Council on Bioethics*, Appendix L (pp. 347–63). Washington, DC: President's Council on Bioethics.

——(2004b) "Potential Use of Cellular Therapy for Patients with Heart Disease," in *Monitoring Stem Cell Research: A Report of the President's Council on Bioethics*, Appendix M (pp. 365–83). Washington, DC: President's Council on Bioethics.

Jaunisch, R. (2004) "The Biology of Nuclear Cloning and the Potential of Embryonic Stem Cells for Transplantation Therapy," in *Monitoring Stem Cell Research: A Report of the President's Council on Bioethics*, Appendix N (pp. 385–414). Washington, DC: President's Council on Bioethics.

Johannes, L. and Regaldo, A. (2004) "Privately Funded Research Yields New Stem-Cell Lines," *The Wall Street Journal*, March 4: B1–2.

Johnson, M. (1995) "Reflections on Some Catholic Claims for Relayed Hominisation," *Theological Studies*, 56: 743–63.

Juengst, E. and Fossel, M. (2000) "The Ethics of Embryonic Stem Cells," *Journal of American Medical Association*, 284: 3180–84.

Kaebnick, G.E. (2001) "Embryonic Stem Cells Without Embryos," *Hastings Center Report*, 31(6): 7.

Kass, L.R. and Wilson, J.Q. (1998) *The Ethics of Human Cloning*, Washington, DC: AEI Press.

Keenan, J. (2001) "Casuistry, Virtue, and the Slippery Slope: Major Problems with Producing Human Embryonic Life for Research Purposes," in P. Lauritzen (ed.) *Cloning and the Future of Human Embryo Research* (pp. 67–81). New York: Oxford University Press.

Keller, G. and Snodgrass, H.R. (1999) "Human Embryonic Stem Cells: The Future is Now," *Nature Medicine*, 5: 151–52.

Kirk, C. (2000) "Research Guidelines: NIH Issues Guidelines for Federally Funded Stem Cell Research," *Journal of Law, Medicine & Ethics*, 28(4): 411–13.

Klotzko, A.J. (2002) "A Cloning Emergency in Britain?," *The Scientist*, 16(1): 12.

Knowles, L.P. (2000/2001) "Science Policy and the Law: Reproductive and Therapeutic Cloning," *New York University School of Law Journal of Legislation and Public Policy*, 4: 13–22.

Lanza, R.P., Caplan, A.L., Silver, L.M., Cibelli, J.B., West, M.D., and Green, R.M. (2000). "The Ethical Validity of Using Nuclear Transfer in Human Transplantation," *Journal of American Medical Association*, 284: 3175–79.

Latham, S. (2002) "Ethics and Politics," *American Journal of Bioethics*, 2(1): 46.

Lauritzen, P. (2004) "Report on the Ethics of Stem Cell Research," in *Monitoring Stem Cell Research: A Report of the President's Council on Bioethics*, Appendix G (pp. 237–72). Washington, DC: President's Council on Bioethics.

——(2001a). "Neither Person nor Property: Embryo Research and the Status of the Early Embryo," *America*, 184(10): 20–23.

——(ed.) (2001b) *Cloning and the Future of Human Embryo Research*, New York: Oxford University Press.

Lebacqz, K., Mendiola, M.M., Peters, T., Young, E.W.D., and Zoloth-Dorfman, L. (Geron Ethics Advisory Board) (1999) "Research with Human Embryonic Stem Cells: Ethical Considerations," *Hastings Center Report*, 29(2): 31–36.

London, A. (2002) "Embryos, Stem Cells, and the 'Strategic' Element in Public Moral Reasoning," *American Journal of Bioethics*, 2(1): 56.

Ludwig, T.E. and Thomson, J.A. (2004) "Current Progress in Human Embryonic Stem Cell Research," in *Monitoring Stem Cell Research: A Report of the President's Council on Bioethics*, Appendix I (pp. 279–94). Washington, DC: President's Council on Bioethics.

Lysaught, M.J. and Hazlehurst, A.L. (2003) "Private Sector Development of Stem Cell Technology and Therapeutic Cloning," *Tissue Engineering*, 9(3): 555–61.

McCartney, J. (2002) "Embryonic Stem Cell Research and Respect for Human Life: Philosophical and Legal Reflections," *Albany Law Review*, 65: 597–624.

McCormick, R.A. (1991) "Who or What is the Preembryo?," *Kennedy Institute of Ethics Journal*, 1: 1–15.

McGee, G. (2002) "The Idolatry of Absolutizing in the Stem Cell Debate," *American Journal of Bioethics*, 2(1): 53–54.

McGee, G. and Caplan, A. (1999) "The Ethics and Politics of Small Sacrifices in Stem Cell Research," *Kennedy Institute of Ethics Journal*, 9: 151–58.

Macklin, R. (1999) "Ethical Problems in Sham Surgery in Clinical Research," *New England Journal of Medicine*, 341(13): 992–96.

Magill, G. (2004) "Science, Ethics, and Policy: Relating Human Genomics with Embryonic Stem Cell Research and Therapeutic Cloning," in G. Magill (ed.) *Genetics and Ethics: An Interdisciplinary Study* (pp. 253–83). St. Louis, MO: Saint Louis University Press.

——(2002) "The Ethics Weave in Human Genomics, Embryonic Stem Cell Research, and Therapeutic Cloning: Promoting and Protecting Society's Interests," *Albany Law Review*, 65(3): 701–28.

Mahowald, M. and Mahowald, A. (2002) "Embryonic Stem Cell Retrieval and a Possible Ethical Bypass," *American Journal of Bioethics*, 2(1): 42–43.

Marshak, D.R., Gardner, R.L., and Gottlieb, D. (eds) (2001) *Stem Cell Biology*, Cold Spring Harbor, NY: Cold Spring Harbor Laboratory Press.

Martin, G.R. (1981) "Isolation of a Pluripotent Cell Line from Early Mouse Embryos Cultured in Medium Conditioned by Teratocarcinoma Cells," *Proceedings of the National Academy of Sciences*, 78: 7634–38.

Martino, R. (2001) "Human Cloning Prohibition Urged," *Origins*, 31: 439–40.

Marwick, C. (1999) "Funding Stem Cell Research," *Journal of American Medical Association*, 281(8): 692–93.

Matthiessen, L. (ed.) (2001) *Survey on Opinions from National Ethics Committees or Similar Bodies: Public Debate and National Legislation in Relation to Human Embryonic Stem Cell Research and Use*, Brussels, Belgium: European Commission Research Directorate General.

Meilander, G. (2001) "The Point of a Ban: Or How to Think about Stem Cell Research," *Hastings Center Report*, 31(1): 9–16.

Meyer, J.R. (2000) "Human Embryonic Stem Cells and Respect for Life," *Journal of Medical Ethics*, 26: 166–70.

Meyer, M.J. and Nelson, L.J. (2001) "Respecting What We Destroy: Reflections on Human Embryo Research," *Hastings Center Report*, 31(1): 16–23.

Mikes, R., OSF (2001) "NBAC and Embryo Ethics," *The National Catholic Bioethics Quarterly*, 1(2): 163–87.

Moreno, J.D. and London, A.J. (2001) "Consensus, Ethics, and Politics in Cloning and Embryo Research," in P. Lauritzen (ed.) *Cloning and the Future of Human Embryo Research* (pp. 162–77). New York: Oxford University Press.

National Bioethics Advisory Commission (NBAC) (2000) *Ethical Issues in Human Stem Cell Research: Vol. II. Commissioned Papers*, Rockville, MD: National Bioethics Advisory Committee.

——(1999) *Ethical Issues in Human Stem Cell Research*, Rockville, MD: National Bioethics Advisory Committee.

——(1997) *Cloning Human Beings: Report and Recommendations of the National Bioethics Advisory Commission*, Rockville, MD: National Bioethics Advisory Committee.

National Commission for the Protection of Human Subjects of Biomedical and Behavioral Research (1975) *Research on the Fetus: Report and Recommendations*, Washington, DC: Department of Health, Education, and Welfare.

National Institutes of Health (NIH) (2005) "Human Embryonic Stem Cell Registry," Online available: http://stemcells.nih.gov/registry/index.asp (accessed July 18, 2005).

——(2001) "Stem Cells: Scientific Progress and Future Research Directions," Online available: http://stemcells.nih.gov/info/scireport/(accessed October 12, 2004).

——(1994a) *Report of the Human Embryo Research Panel*, Bethesda, MD: National Institutes of Health.

——(1994b) *Papers Commissioned for the Human Embryo Research Panels*, 2 vols, Bethesda, MD: National Institutes of Health.

National Research Council, Institute of Medicine (NRC/IOM) (2001/2002) *Stem Cells and the Future of Regenerative Medicine*, Washington, DC: National Academies Press.

Noonan, J.T., Jr (1973) "Raw Judicial Power," *National Review*, 25(9): 260–64.

"Open Letter to President Bush Regarding Council on Bioethics" (2004) *American Journal of Bioethics*, Online available: http://bioethics.net/openletter.php (9 March 2003) (accessed April 10, 2004).

Orr, R. (2002) "The Moral Status of the Embryonic Stem Cell: Inherent or Imputed?," *American Journal of Bioethics*, 2(1): 57–59.

Outka, Gene (2002) "The Ethics of Stem Cell Research," *Kennedy Institute of Ethics Journal*, 12(2): 175–213.

Parker, S.M. (2001) "Bringing the 'Gospel of Life' to American Jurisprudence: A Religious, Ethical, and Philosophical Critique of Federal Funding for Embryonic Stem Cell Research," *Journal of Contemporary Health Law and Policy*, 17: 771–808.

Pennings, G., Schots, R., and Liebaers, I. (2002) "Ethical Considerations on Preimplantation Genetic Diagnosis for HLA Typing to Match a Future Child as a Donor of Haematopoietic Stem Cells to a Sibling," *Human Reproduction*, 17(3): 534–38.

Phimister, E.G. and Drazen, J.M. (2004) "Two Fillips for Human Embryonic Stem Cells," *New England Journal of Medicine*, 350(13): 1351–52.

Porter, J. (1995) "Individuality, Personal Identity, and the Moral Status of the Preembryo: A Response to Mark Johnson," *Theological Studies*, 56: 763–70.

Prentice, D.A. (2004) "Adult Stem Cells," in *Monitoring Stem Cell Research: A Report of the President's Council on Bioethics*, Appendix K (pp. 309–46). Washington, DC: President's Council on Bioethics.

President's Council on Bioethics (2004) *Monitoring Stem Cell Research: A Report of the President's Council on Bioethics*, Washington, DC: President's Council on Bioethics.

——(2002) *Human Cloning and Human Dignity: The Report of the President's Council on Bioethics*, New York: Public Affairs.

Rainey, E.R. and Magill, G. (1996) *Abortion & Public Policy*, Omaha, Nebraska: Creighton University Press.

Resnik, D. (2002) "The Commercialization of Human Stem Cells: Ethical and Policy Issues," *Health Care Analysis*, 10: 127–54.

Robertson, J. (2003a) "Extending Preimplantation Genetic Diagnosis: The Ethical Debate: Ethical Issues in New Uses of Preimplantation Genetic Diagnosis," *Human Reproduction*, 18: 465–71.

——(2003b) "Extending Preimplantation Genetic Diagnosis: Medical and Non-Medical Uses," *Journal of Medical Ethics*, 29: 213–16.

Robertson, J. (1999) "Ethics and Policy in Embryonic Stem Cell Research," *Kennedy Institute of Ethics Journal*, 9(2): 109–36.

Robertson, J., Kahn, J., and Wagner, J. (2002) "Conception to Obtain Haematopoietic Stem Cells," *Hastings Center Report*, 32(3): 34–40.

Roe v. Wade 410 US 113 (1973).

Romeo-Casabona, C.M. (2002) "Embryonic Stem Cell Research and Therapy: The Need for a Common European Legal Framework," *Bioethics*, 16(6): 557–67.

Rosso, E. (1999) "A Look Back at NBAC," *The Scientist*, 13(20): 4.

Royal Commission on New Reproductive Technologies (1993) *Proceed with Care: Report of the Royal Commission on New Reproductive Technologies*, Ottowa, Canada: Ministry of Government Services.

Ryan, M.A. (2001) "Creating Embryos for Research: On Weighing Symbolic Costs," in P. Lauritzen (ed.) *Cloning and the Future of Human Embryo Research* (pp. 50–66). New York: Oxford University Press.

Savulescu, J. (2002) "The Embryonic Stem Cell Lottery and the Cannibalization of Human Beings," *Bioethics*, 16(6): 508–29.

Scott, W.K., Nance, M.A., Watts, R.L., Hubble, J.P., Koller, W.C., Lyons, K., Pahwa, R., Stern, M.B., Colcher, A., Hiner, B.C., Jankovic, J., Ondo, W.G., Allen, F.H., Jr, Goetz, C.G., Small, G.W., Masterman, D., Mastaglia, F., Laing, N.G., Stajich, J.M., Slotterbeck, B., Booze, M.W., Ribble, R.C., Rampersaud, E., West, S.G., Gibson, R.A., Middleton, L.T., Roses, A.D., Haines, J.L., Scott, B.L., Vance, J.M., and Pericak-Vanceet, M.A. (2001) "Complete Genomic Screen in Parkinson Disease: Evidence for Multiple Genes," *Journal of American Medical Association*, 286: 2239–44.

Shamblot, M.J., Axelman, J., Wang, S., Bugg, E.M., Littlefield, J.W., Donovan, P.J., Blumenthal, P.D., Huggins, G.R., and Gearhart, J.D. (1998) "Derivation of Human Pluripotent Stem Cells from Cultured Primordial Germ Cells," *Proceedings of the National Academy of Sciences*, 95(23): 13726–31.

Shannon, T.A. (2002) "Human Cloning," *America*, 186(5): 15–18.

——(1997) "Fetal Status: Sources and Implications," *Journal of Medicine and Philosophy*, 22: 415–22.

Shannon, T. and Wolter, A.B. (1990) "Reflections on the Moral Status of the Pre-Embryo," *Theological Studies*, 51: 603–26.

Shapiro, R.S. (2003) "Legislative Research Bans on Human Cloning," *Cambridge Quarterly of Healthcare Ethics*, 12: 393–400.

Sleator, A. (2000) *Stem Cell Research and Regulations under the Human Fertilisation and Embryology Act 1990*. December 13. London: House of Commons.

Solbakk, J.J. (2003) "Use and Abuse of Empirical Knowledge in Contemporary Bioethics: A Critical Analysis of Empirical Arguments Employed in the Controversy Surrounding Stem Cell Research," *Cambridge Quarterly of Healthcare Ethics*, 12: 384–92.

Spike, J. (2003) "Bush and Stem Cell Research: An Ethically Confused Policy," *American Journal of Bioethics*, 2(1): 46.

Steinberg, D. (2002) "Can Moral Worthiness Be Seen Using a Microscope?," *American Journal of Bioethics*, 2(1): 49.

Steinbock, B. (2001) "Respect for Human Embryos," in P. Lauritzen (ed.) *Cloning and the Future of Human Embryo Research* (pp. 21–33). New York: Oxford University Press.

——(1992) *Life before Birth: The Moral and Legal Status of Embryos and Fetuses*, New York: Oxford University Press.

Stiltner, B. (2001) "Morality, Religion, and Public Bioethics: Shifting the Paradigm for the Public Discussion of Embryo Research and Human Cloning," in P. Lauritzen (ed.) *Cloning and the Future of Human Embryo Research* (pp. 178–200). New York: Oxford University Press.

Strong, C. (1997) "The Moral Status of Preembryos, Embryos, Fetuses, and Infants," *The Journal of Medicine and Philosophy*, 22(5): 457–58.

Suarez, A. (1990) "Hydatidiform Moles and Teratomas Confirm the Human Identity of the Preimplantation Embryo," *Journal of Medicine and Philosophy*, 1: 630–36.

Sullivan, D. (2003) "The Conception View of Personhood: A Review," *Ethics and Medicine*. 19(1): 11–33.

"Symposium: Human Primordial Stem Cells." (1999) *Hastings Center Report*, 29(2): 30–48.

Tauer, C.A. (2001) "Responsibility and Regulation: Reproductive Technologies, Cloning, and Embryo Research," in P. Lauritzen (ed.) *Cloning and the Future of Human Embryo Research* (pp. 145–61). New York: Oxford University Press.

——(1997) "Embryo Research and Public Policy," *Journal of Medicine and Philosophy*, 22: 423–39.

Thomson, J.A., Itskovitz-Eldor, J., Shapiro, S.S., Waknitz, M.A., Swiergiel, J.J., Marshall, V.S., and Jones, J.M. (1998) "Embryonic Stem Cell Lines Derived from Human Blastocysts," *Science*, 282: 1145–47 [erratum, *Science*, 282 (1998): 1827].

Towner, D. and Loewy, R.S. (2002) "Ethics of Preimplantation Diagnosis for a Woman Destined to Develop Early-Onset Alzheimer Disease," *Journal of American Medical Association*, 287: 1038–40.

Tribe, L.H. (1988) *American Constitutional Law*, Mineola, NY: The Foundation Press.

UK Department of Health (2002) *Stem Cell Research Report from the Select Committee*, London: Her Majesty's Stationery Office.

——(2000) *Stem Cell Research: Medical Progress with Responsibility. A Report from the Chief Medical Officer's Expert Group Reviewing the Potential of Developments in Stem Cell Research and Cell Nuclear Replacement to Benefit Human Health*, August, London: Her Majesty's Stationery Office. Online available: http://www.doh.gov.uk/cegs/stemcellreport.htm (accessed October 12, 2004).

Verfaillie, C.M. (2004) "Multipotent Adult Progenitor Cells: An Update," in *Monitoring Stem Cell Research: A Report of the President's Council on Bioethics*, Appendix J (pp. 295–307). Washington, DC: President's Council on Bioethics.

Verlinsky, Y., Rechitsky, S., Schoolcraft, W., Strom, C., and Kuliev, A. (2001) "Preimplantation Diagnosis for Fanconi Anemia Combined with HLA Matching," *Journal of American Medical Association*, 285: 3130–33.

Walters, L. (2004) "The United Nations and Human Cloning: A Debate on Hold," *Hastings Center Report* 34(1): 5–6.

Warnock, M. (1985a) *A Question of Life: The Warnock Report on Fertilisation and Embryology*. Oxford: Basil Blackwell.

——(1985b) "The Warnock Report," *British Medical Journal*, 291: 187–89.

Weissman, I.L. (2002) "Stem Cells—Scientific, Medical, and Political Issues," *New England Journal of Medicine*, 346(20): 1576–79.

Wildes, K.W. (1999) "The Stem Cell Report," *America*, 181(11): 12–14.

Wilkie, D. (2004) "Stealth Stipulation Shadows Stem Cell Research," *The Scientist*, 18(4): 42–43.

Willgoos, C. (2001) "FDA Regulation: An Answer to the Questions of Human Cloning and Germline Gene Therapy," *American Journal of Law & Medicine*, 27: 101–24.

Wilmut, I. (1998) "Cloning for Medicine," *Scientific American*, 279 (December): 58–63.

Wilmut, I. and Schnieke, A.E. (1997) "Viable Offspring Derived from Fetal and Adult Mammalian Cells," *Nature*, 385(6619): 810–13.

Wolf, S.M., Kahn, J.P., and Wagner, J.E. (2003) "Using Preimplantation Genetic Diagnosis to Create a Stem Cell Donor: Issues, Guidelines, and Limits," *Journal of Law, Medicine & Ethics*, 31: 327–39.

5 Conducting and terminating randomized controlled trials

Ana Smith Iltis

Research and experimentation are the avenues through which physicians can determine which interventions are more likely than not to benefit patients overall. As such, research is a necessary condition for enabling physicians in the future to execute the therapeutic obligation and the obligation of beneficence. Some research consists of retrospective or observational studies in which the conduct of research does not affect patients' treatment decisions. But often it involves the randomization of patients to different interventions and the prospective assessment of outcomes. Patients are simultaneously patients and subjects, hereafter referred to as patient-subjects, and decisions regarding the interventions they receive are determined by chance.[1] The circumstances under which it is ethically permissible for physicians to conduct such randomized controlled trials (RCTs) and when those RCTs may include a placebo arm (placebo controlled trials or PCTs) have received significant attention in the medical and research ethics literature as well as, from time to time, the popular press.[2] At its core, the debate concerns the tension between the commitments and obligations of persons who are both clinicians and researchers. The commitment to conduct biomedical research that will yield useful data and scientifically valid results generates a set of obligations that may, at times, conflict with clinicians' obligations. To fulfill their therapeutic obligation and their obligation of beneficence, clinicians are expected to protect and respect the interests of individual patients. Researchers are expected to protect the rights and safety of subjects while conducting investigations that will make it possible to respond to patient-subjects' interests in the future and/or to the interests of other patients in the future. RCTs often are used to eliminate or minimize bias in assessing which treatments, overall, are best. Yet, the commitment to individual patients requires physicians to recommend interventions to persons based on what is expected to be best for them given their circumstances. The use of placebos raises special concerns because in PCTs some patient-subjects receive no intervention for their medical condition. This chapter offers an overview of the principal ethical issues concerning RCTs and PCTs: (1) when is it permissible to conduct an RCT? (2) when is it permissible to conduct an RCT in which at least some subjects will be randomized to placebo? (3) when ought an RCT be stopped?

Assessing randomization: the permissibility of randomized controlled trials

A significant number of contributors to the research ethics literature hold that when research is being conducted on patient-subjects (persons who are entering a trial designed to assess treatments for a condition the subjects have), the obligations physicians have to attempt to do what is in a patient's best interests must remain the principal basis for a physician's actions and recommendations.[3] The goals of research may not trump the goals of clinical care when subjects also are patients, and physicians ought not to invite their patients to join trials that they think conflict with their patients' interest (Freedman 1987; Giesen 1995; Kodish *et al.* 1991; Levine 1985, 1986; World Medical Association 2000). If this is the case, then physicians generally should recommend to patients whatever interventions they have reason to believe will be overall best for their patients. Only when there is equipoise, that is, when there is genuine uncertainty as to whether one treatment is likely to be better overall than another treatment, is it permissible for physicians to conduct RCTs on patient-subjects.

Some have argued that there is a moral difference between the obligations of clinical and research medicine, and that researchers do not possess the obligation of beneficence, and the therapeutic obligation we attribute to clinicians. For example, Miller and Brody argue:

> Physicians in clinical practice have a duty to promote the medical best interests of patients by offering optimal medical care. In RCTs, however, physician-investigators are not offering personalized medical therapy for individual patients. Rather, they seek to answer clinically relevant scientific questions by conducting experiments that test the safety and efficacy of treatments in groups of patients. The process of treatment in RCTs differs radically from routine clinical practice. ... Owing to these fundamental differences in purpose and process, the ethics of clinical trials is not identical to the ethics of clinical medicine. Specifically, the obligations of physician-investigators are not the same as the obligations of physicians in routine clinical practice. Investigators have a duty to avoid exploiting research participants, not a therapeutic duty to provide optimal medical care.
>
> (2002: 4–5)

They make a similar argument in Miller and Brody (2003). Miller and Brody's position has merit as they articulate it. Clinical and research medicine are different endeavors with different goals, and clinicians and researchers have different obligations. However, the structure of the research environment at present is such that often subjects are patients and remain patients throughout the course of a study, in both their own minds and from the perspective of their physicians. When the line between research medicine and clinical medicine cannot be drawn sharply, a strong case can be made for insisting that clinician-researchers continue to be obligated toward their patients as clinicians. One could respond that any time a patient enrolls in a trial, that person becomes a subject, not a patient-subject. The line between research and clinical medicine can and should be drawn more clearly. Rather than focusing on how clinicians can satisfy their obligations while conducting research, we should turn our attention to improving informed consent. In all matters related to the trial, the investigator's obligation is to protect that subject's rights and welfare in the research process, but not to act in that person's best clinical interests. Anyone who insists otherwise suffers from the therapeutic misconception and the requirement for equipoise perpetuates this misconception.[4] One also could suggest, as Miller and Brody (2002) do, that clinicians should not enroll their own patients in (some) RCTs. But this is difficult to envision in the current research environment.

One can imagine an environment in which the lines between research and clinical medicine are clearer, as Rebecca Dresser (2002) does in considering ways to reduce the therapeutic misconception. But the current methods for recruiting subjects into research and the circumstance that research is conducted in the clinical context make it virtually impossible to proceed as if the line between research and clinical medicine always is clear. This chapter focuses on RCTs involving patient-subjects, for whom the line between clinical care and research is "fuzzy." In those cases, clinician-researchers may understandably see themselves as having an obligation to act in the interests of their patients, and patient-subjects may have a claim on investigators to do so.

A number of authors have proposed the requirement of equipoise as a necessary condition for conducting RCTs, at least in the case of patient-subjects. However, there is no universal agreement that equipoise is a necessary condition to conduct trials or that it is a coherent concept (Ashcroft 1999). Deborah Hellman (2002), for example, has argued that the concept of equipoise is not capable of addressing the tension that exists between clinicians' and researchers' obligations. Following statistician Richard Royall (1997), she distinguishes three questions: What does the evidence show? Given the evidence, what should I believe? Given the evidence, what should I do? Equipoise involves beliefs; one is in equipoise because one is unsure, given the evidence, what one should believe. For clinicians and for patients, the most important question is not "What should I believe?" but "What should I do?" That there is uncertainty of belief, she argues, does not mean that there is or should be uncertainty about how to act. Despite criticism of the concept, the term "equipoise" is widely used in offering justifications for RCTs and has played an important role in the research ethics literature for the last three decades.

Even among those who agree on the importance of uncertainty in justifying RCTs, the locus of the uncertainty has been and continues to be debated. One may hold, as did Charles Fried (1974), that it is permissible to enroll patients into RCTs when there is no evidence that one intervention is superior to another. But, as numerous authors have pointed out, if there were an absolute state of uncertainty (50–50 percent), we would not think a clinical trial was justifiable or necessary in the first place. Clinical trials are designed to assess evidence already gathered that one intervention may be better than another.[5] This form of equipoise has since been called "theoretical equipoise," referring to its focus on a precise degree of uncertainty regarding two interventions (Freedman 1987). The principal difficulties attributed to it relate to the "knife's edge" precision it requires. First, it will (almost) never be possible to justify in principle starting a clinical trial if a precise 50–50 balance of uncertainty must exist, that is, if there must be no evidence at all that one is better than the other. Second, any amount of evidence that becomes available may disturb the balance, making it impermissible to continue a RCT. Any clinician who perceives the evidence as not being precisely balanced will find it unacceptable to enroll patients in the first place. One who perceives a shift in the balance will be unable to continue to enroll patients in a trial that once was justifiable, and subjects already enrolled will have to be withdrawn. Freedman attempted to reformulate equipoise in a way that would avoid the knife's edge precision Fried's equipoise seems to require. "Clinical equipoise" exists when "[t]here is no consensus within the expert clinical community about the comparative merits of the alternatives to be tested" (1987: 144). The character of the consensus is open to question. Are RCTs permissible as long as some clinician disagrees with another clinician, or must there be a fairly even division of opinion? Lack of consensus could be achieved with only one dissenter, but this is not likely to be the ethical basis for rendering randomization permissible.[6]

Although Freedman and others have applied this principle to argue against the permissibility of many trials, especially PCTs, it was developed in part in an effort to refine Fried's conception of theoretical equipoise in a way that would promote medical research. During the 1970s and early 1980s it became apparent that when physicians abided by Fried's standard, many of them did not enroll patients into clinical trials and research progressed slowly. Individual clinicians who felt that there was evidence that one treatment was better (even if only slightly better) than the other were unwilling to enroll patients. The refusal to enroll patients into RCTs did not reflect consensus or even substantial agreement in the medical community regarding the superiority of one intervention or another, however. Some clinicians favored one intervention and some favored another. Uncertainty remained within the medical community, and without research there would be no advance in knowledge. Yet, following the theoretical equipoise model made it impossible to conduct research to the point of statistical significance because any evidence favoring one or the other made enrollment in RCTs impermissible.[7] Freedman argued that a model grounded in a more general uncertainty or disagreement in the clinical community would support medical research more reliably. Even if an individual clinician thought that there was some evidence that one treatment was better than another, he could defer to the lack of consensus in the clinical community and enroll patients in an RCT.

Both Fried and Freedman held that the medical community is the source of medical knowledge and the judge of what constitutes sound practice. Yet, one must assess who constitutes the relevant medical community. Is it genuine uncertainty among experts in a given field, as Freedman asserts (1987: 144), or among a broader community of clinicians? Here, Fred Gifford (1995) observes, advocates of clinical equipoise offer conflicting responses depending on their rationale for supporting clinical equipoise as the relevant standard. If one relies on what Gifford calls the "evidential warrant rationale" for clinical equipoise, a clinician recognizes disagreement among experts as calling into question his previous preference for one treatment over another. On the other hand, if one supports the concept of clinical equipoise on the "they're no worse of than they would otherwise have been rationale," one will identify physicians more broadly as the relevant medical community. It is permissible to conduct an RCT if patient-subjects are expected to end up no worse off than they would have had they not enrolled in the trial. If there is uncertainty in the medical community at large regarding the superiority of one treatment or another, then even among those who do not enroll in an RCT, some will receive one treatment and some the other. This is precisely what will occur in an RCT, and thus those in the RCT are expected to end up no worse off than those not in the RCT.[8]

The conceptions of equipoise discussed thus far emphasize the importance of uncertainty among (at least) some members of the community because medical knowledge is social in nature.[9] Others have suggested that medical knowledge is grounded not only in the medical community but also in the lay or patient community such that "community equipoise" is necessary to justify RCTs. Jason Karlawish and John Lantos, for example, argue for community equipoise in part because they view it as a mechanism for accounting for patients' values in assessing treatments (1997: 388) and in part because they hold that both physicians' and patients' judgments together constitute medical knowledge: "medical knowledge is not confined to the profession of physicians. Instead, the community of physicians and patients constructs the judgment that their collective uncertainty justifies a trial and the kind of trial it justifies" (1997: 387). They argue that "[t]o the same extent that physician and patient values should govern clinical decisionmaking, they should govern research decisionmaking according to a process called shared decisionmaking" (1997: 386). Only when the clinical community and patients as a whole believe an RCT is justifiable should it be deemed permissible. The claim regarding shared decision-making in both the clinical and research setting is valid, but it supports only the importance of taking into account a patient's values in making clinical treatment decisions and research participation decisions with individual patients. The phrase "[t]o the same extent" suggests a conflation of decision-making regarding individual patients with decisions regarding patients in general. The clinical community does not consult with patients to assess whether patients agree with what clinicians think should be standard of care or what clinical guidelines should be followed. The expectation is that decisions regarding whether a particular patient will receive the standard of care are made by patients and physicians together, but that does not change physicians' general recommendations.

This is not to say that patients' values are irrelevant to the research process. They are central to assessing whether it is permissible to randomize a specific patient. And there may be pragmatic reasons to include some patients in designing studies and developing recruitment strategies so as to ensure adequate enrollment and enhance subjects' willingness to remain in a study. But what one person considers impermissible or a risk not worth taking, another may be willing or even happy to volunteer to do. As long as some patients are willing to enroll in an RCT, and there appears to be a legitimate research question, there seems to be no reason to require that patients as a whole be in equipoise. We need not require that approximately half of all patients think the research question is worth answering in an RCT. Nor need we require that all or most patients be in equipoise regarding a treatment preference.

Community equipoise would require that one or the other of the conditions be fulfilled. Patients' willingness to enroll in studies is most appropriately assessed in the informed consent stage of research, not at the stage of determining whether a trial is in principle permissible. To establish whether community equipoise exists, one must determine who the relevant patients are and why their values ought to govern research, be able to identify the beliefs of those patients reliably, determine how knowledgeable they must be for their beliefs to be considered in assessing research options, and assess how patients' beliefs and the beliefs of the clinical community will be balanced.[10]

With these caveats in mind, some form of community equipoise might be appropriate in assessing whether RCTs that must be conducted without informed consent, such as some emergency treatment protocols, are in principle permissible. When it is not possible to seek consent, the decision that it is in principle permissible to conduct an RCT cannot be fully separated from decisions regarding the permissibility of randomizing specific patients. Without informed consent, a person's values and beliefs cannot be considered in assessing whether randomization is acceptable to that patient. In those cases, it may be necessary, or at least appropriate, to include the opinions of the lay public at the preliminary stage of determining the in-principle permissibility of conducting an RCT even though no perfectly representative sample exists and there is no substitute for the values and preferences of individual patients. The difficulties associated with knowing what patients believe, managing conflicts among patients' values and beliefs, and so on remain, but we may accept those limitations and pursue community opinion because there may be no other opportunity to consider patients' values.[11] The reliance on community equipoise should not be understood as implying that consent can be replaced by community opinion. We defer to community equipoise in such cases because the character of some emergency research precludes informed consent, making it impossible to include patients' values and preferences in determining research participation. Yet, we desire to consider patients' values, insofar as possible, in assessing the permissibility of entering them into an RCT. In protocols in which informed consent cannot be obtained because of the nature of the study, community equipoise may be useful in judging the in-principle permissibility of a trial.

In addition to recognizing equipoise as a necessary condition for rendering RCTs in principle permissible, some have argued that the interventions being tested in the RCT also must be available outside the research context to justify an RCT (Kodish *et al.* 1991). There may be cases in which a clinician, patient, or both have a preference for one treatment over another, but the intervention preferred is not available outside the context of an RCT. Physicians may offer or even recommend participation in an RCT, and patients may seek or accept enrollment in a trial in order to have the chance of accessing the desired intervention. In those cases, physicians and/or patients do not actually want to participate in an RCT, but they pursue research participation to try to access a particular intervention. Unless the interventions being studied in the RCT also are available outside the RCT, randomization is unethical because patients may feel that they must participate in research and physicians may not be free to offer individual patients the treatments they think are most appropriate for them (Kodish *et al.* 1991).

One should neither dismiss too quickly nor underestimate the possible costs of insisting that RCTs be conducted only when the interventions being tested are also available outside the context of RCTs. There are examples in recent medical history in which some physicians and patients strongly favored one intervention over another. They did not accept the circumstance that the intervention had not been proven safe or effective, as grounds for either not pursuing it at all or participating in an RCT in which they might or might not receive it. Yet, when the intervention finally was studied in RCTs, it was found to be ineffective or harmful (or both). The culture of assuming that the latest interventions always are better can contribute to a sense that RCTs are unacceptable and to a demand for access to new interventions prior to and outside the context of RCTs. The rationale is not always irrational: persons with conditions that are likely to be severely debilitating or fatal before the results of an RCT are available believe that it is worth trying anything. But this belief can harm not only those patients who use the experimental interventions but other patients in the future who cannot benefit from the knowledge gained in RCTs. Moreover, they can drain social resources by directing health-care resources toward what may be ineffective interventions and they leave physicians to act in ways that conflict with the obligation of beneficence.

There are numerous examples of this phenomenon, one of the most notable of which comes from the world of breast cancer research. In the mid-1980s, it was thought that women with advanced breast cancer might be treated with high-dose chemotherapy and bone marrow transplants. When the experimental treatment was first used in advanced breast cancer patients, 15–20 percent of the patients died as a result of the interventions (Dresser 2001: 62). There was little interest in participating in RCTs, not because of these deaths, but because patients did not want to risk being assigned to the standard treatment arm. Physicians and hospitals often were willing to provide the experimental intervention outside the RCT context. Even though insurers were largely unwilling to pay for the experimental procedures, threats of lawsuits often resulted in coverage. It took nearly fifteen years to conduct RCTs comparing standard treatment to high-dose chemotherapy with bone marrow transplantation, and the RCTs showed that the experimental intervention was not any better than the standard treatment (Burgh 2000; Dresser 2001: 62). In the meantime, many people had undergone painful procedures for no benefit and either spent large amounts of money from their own pockets to pay for treatment or used social resources to pay for experimental interventions. It is not difficult to find counterexamples, cases in which a significant number of patients wanted access to an experimental intervention outside the context of RCTs and the intervention turned out to be superior. But we can only determine whether both patients' and clinicians' preferences were "right" after the fact. The chances of "getting it wrong" are real, and the costs to both current and future patients, as well as to society, can be high. At the very least, we should give serious consideration to attempting to determine when research is in principle necessary and randomization in principle permissible through what amounts to opinion polls among a wide range of clinicians and patients, many of whom may be poorly informed, and we should consider carefully the costs of requiring that experimental interventions be available outside the context of RCTs as a necessary condition for rendering such trials permissible.

Scholarship on the ethics of randomizing patient-subjects continues to grow and there is no agreement on which understanding of equipoise, if any, must be met to justify RCTs. Despite the disagreements, the word "equipoise" is routinely used by investigators attempting to justify RCTs and institutional review board (IRB) members deliberating the permissibility of particular RCTs. But because there is no single understanding of equipoise and no objective measure of its existence, judgments regarding the importance of answering the research question and the risks associated with randomization may play a greater role in those justifications and deliberations than any particular conception of equipoise.

Even if one relies on some conception of equipoise as a basis for justifying in principle the initiation of an RCT, that equipoise may not exist throughout the course of a trial. As preliminary data become available, the uncertainty clinicians and/or patients once experienced may no longer exist. Although the data may not be sufficient to yield statistical significance, they may be sufficient to disturb equipoise.[12] Thus the initial in-principle permissibility of an RCT may not sustain its permissibility throughout its duration. At some point during the trial it may become in principle impermissible to randomize more patient-subjects or to ask currently enrolled subjects to remain in the trial. Thus, even if an RCT is in principle permissible at one time, as the trial progresses it may no longer be justifiable on the same grounds that rendered its initiation justified. The issue of assessing during the course of a trial whether it should be stopped because statistical significance has been reached, because there are serious safety concerns, or because there is evidence that one treatment is superior even though the evidence is not statistically significant, is discussed in the final section of this chapter.

Placebo controlled trials

Many of the concerns that emerge in the debate regarding the ethics of RCTs are magnified when those trials involve the comparison of an intervention with placebo. Benjamin Freedman, whose work on clinical equipoise has shaped the research ethics literature, argued that "placebo is ethical only in investigations for conditions for which there is no known treatment" (1987: 141). Active controlled trials (ACTs) should be conducted in all other cases (and only when equipoise exists between all arms of the study). This view is reflected in the Declaration of Helsinki (WMA 2000, 2002), though those guidelines permit exceptions for new interventions designed to treat "a minor condition and the patients who receive placebo will not be subject to any additional risk of serious or irreversible harm" and for situations in which there are "compelling and scientifically sound methodological reasons" for conducting a PCT (WMA 2002). The argument that to conduct PCTs when an established therapy exists is a violation of physicians' therapeutic obligation and obligation of beneficence has been articulated by a number of authors (e.g., Freedman 1987; Freedman *et al.* 1996a,b; Lemmens and Miller 2002). In these cases, consent is insufficient and physicians ought not to raise the possibility of participation in a PCT with patients. These objections have been criticized by some (e.g., Miller and Brody 2002; Veatch 2002a,b), and some have argued that they may restrict the permissibility of PCTs but not altogether prohibit them (e.g., Iltis 2004). Some who object to the use of PCTs whenever there is an established therapy also object to the use of PCTs when "pretrial clinical evidence" indicates that a new intervention may be effective (Glass and Waring 2002: 26). Depending on how broadly one interprets the signs of efficacy from pretrial clinical evidence, PCTs may never be permissible. Nor for that matter may most ACTs be permissible, since the reason for testing a new intervention in clinical trials is that there already is some evidence that it may be effective. Without those early indications, one would consider a clinical trial inappropriate. It is not at all clear how the obligation to offer patients experimental interventions is equivalent to the obligation to offer them standard care, yet the basis for this argument is that offering experimental interventions is a product of physicians' therapeutic obligation. The costs of pursuing these restrictions on the research process may be high for both patient-subjects enrolled in ACTs and future patients.

Some have suggested that PCTs are not only unethical but also not scientifically necessary when there already is an established treatment for the condition a new intervention is designed to treat (Freedman *et al.* 1996b; Rothman and Michels 1994). When an established treatment already exists, they argue, the scientific question investigators ought to ask is whether the new intervention is better than the established one, not better than nothing, which is what a PCT would tell us. Others have argued that we should not be so confident in the scientific superiority of ACTs or even in the power of ACTs to provide data that are as reliable and useful as PCTs (Temple and Ellenberg 2000a,b). ACTs may require more subjects and time, and it may take longer for safety concerns to emerge, for example. Thus, more patient-subjects may be enrolled, and they may be enrolled as subjects for longer than they otherwise would have been. Moreover, in studies designed to test interventions for conditions with a high rate of placebo response, results of ACTs may not show that a new intervention actually is better than nothing (Emanuel and Miller 2001). Even for conditions that do not have a high rate of placebo response, there are design factors that sometimes make ACTs more likely than PCTs to show false positives (Hart 1999). As a result, patients may use drugs that are not medically necessary, exposing them to unnecessary risks and side effects, and personal and social resources may be directed at paying for unnecessary interventions.

Monitoring and stopping RCTs

Medical research has the ultimate purpose of shaping clinical practice and enabling physicians to offer their patients treatments that overall are better for them. To do that, research must be conducted in such a way that studies yield reliable and useful assessments of interventions, which requires that they be conducted in a sufficiently unbiased manner, for a sufficient period of time and with a large enough number of subjects to achieve statistical significance. At the same time, there is an interest in making better interventions available sooner rather than later and in not exposing persons to the risks and burdens associated with research for longer than necessary. Hence, there is an interest in stopping trials as soon as is appropriate. For all these reasons, choosing the endpoints of a study, the parameters the study will be designed to measure, as well as decisions of when to stop trials are important and involve judgments about facts, values, and interests (Brody 1998: 155–59). Because medical interventions typically are designed to decrease morbidity or mortality, one might expect that a trial's endpoint would be a decrease in the relevant morbidity or mortality among patients. There are cases in which comparing the impact different interventions have on morbidity or mortality may take a long time and/or may require a very large number of subjects. In the interest of assessing the efficacy of new interventions over a shorter period of time or with fewer subjects, sometimes surrogate endpoints are chosen. Surrogate endpoints are endpoints closely correlated to the clinically relevant endpoints (usually a decrease in morbidity or mortality) that can serve as reliable indications that an intervention will have the intended clinical benefits (Brody 1998: 180). A study is designed to measure whether the intervention affects a prognostic marker, or a set of markers, rather than whether it actually decreases morbidity or mortality over the long term. The goal is to choose a surrogate endpoint that correlates with the desired reduction in morbidity or mortality but that can be measured earlier and with fewer subjects than one could measure the clinically relevant endpoint. For example, an antiretroviral drug to treat human immunodeficiency virus (HIV) infection is aimed at reducing the development of acquired immunodeficiency syndrome (AIDS) and death in HIV-positive patients. But the drug's efficacy may be assessed using a surrogate endpoint, such as time to loss of virological control. The issue of how robust the correlation between the surrogate endpoint and the clinically relevant endpoints remains controversial because surrogate endpoints do not always accurately measure an intervention's capacity to lead to the clinically relevant endpoints.[13]

Whether or not surrogate endpoints are used, interim data from clinical trials typically is monitored, sometimes by an independent committee (such as a data safety monitoring board or DSMB), to determine whether (1) the accepted stopping rules for trials indicate that a level of statistical significance has been achieved,[14] (2) the evidence strongly points to the effectiveness of one intervention and the benefit is sufficiently important to warrant an early stop even though statistical significance has not been achieved, (3) there are safety concerns that warrant stopping a trial, or (4) data from other trials alone or together with data from the trial in question suggest a treatment is effective or that there are serious safety concerns. Monitoring trials and making decisions about when to stop them has been described as an ethical balancing act:

> The basic ethical conflict in monitoring trial results is to balance the interest of patients within the trial—that is, the individual ethics of randomizing the next patient—and the longer term interest of obtaining reliable conclusions on sufficient data—that is, the collective ethics of making appropriate treatment policies for future patients.
>
> (Pocock 1992: 235)

To stop a trial early can have costs. For example, long-term safety problems may not have emerged when the trial is stopped and it may take longer to identify those concerns outside the research context. Or, an intervention that is effective in the short term may not be effective over longer periods of time. These difficulties can be managed, in part, through follow-up studies.[15] Moreover, a treatment that may be highly effective may not be adopted by the medical community as standard of practice because there may be doubts about the significance of the evidence that suggests its superiority. This lack of credibility is a significant concern, since the goal of research is to improve practice and care in the future, and the importance of improving treatment options typically plays a role in justifying exposing patient-subjects to risk (Pocock 1999). At the same time, failure to stop a trial early can result in unjustifiable research, unnecessary delays in treatment, and exposure of patient-subjects to unnecessary risks.

There may be times when interim data are not sufficient to stop a trial but might be of interest to enrolled subjects and might affect the willingness of some subjects to continue in the trial. Because informed consent is a process that continues after a person enrolls in a trial rather than an event that occurs prior to enrollment, and because subjects typically are told that they will be provided with any new information that emerges during the course of the trial that may affect their willingness to participate, information from interim data analyses may be reported to patient-subjects. This information may lead some to withdraw from a study. There is a concern that if too many people withdraw from a study, it will not be possible to continue a trial. The goal, then, is to identify what information actually should be provided to patient-subjects and what information is too preliminary so as not to constitute a significant finding that should be reported. There is an interest in preventing patient-subjects from rushing to judgment based on scant information, thus making it impossible to compare interventions. At the same time, patient-subjects' right to important new information should not be compromised.

The discussion of stopping trials early here has focused on ethical and statistical justifications for such decisions. A growing area of controversy in recent years has been decisions by industry sponsors to stop trials early for commercial reasons. A discussion of this issue is beyond the scope of this chapter. For further discussion, see Ashcroft (2001), Boyd (2001), Evans and Pocock (2001), Lièvre *et al.* (2001), Psaty and Rennie (2003), Viberti *et al.* (1997).

The complexity of the concerns surrounding decisions to conduct randomized controlled trials, including placebo controlled trials, assessments of clinicians' and researchers' roles, decisions regarding the endpoints to be used in assessing new interventions, and judgments of when trials should be discontinued prior to reaching those endpoints, suggests that the debate is likely to continue.

Notes

1 Although we typically refer to the randomization of individuals, some studies involve "cluster randomization." Groups of persons, such as members of a community or school, are randomized. A study might be conducted, for example, to assess whether a fitness program in a school is effective in reducing risk factors for diabetes in children. Some schools might be randomized to participate in the fitness program and others would not, serving as controls. For further discussion of cluster randomization, see Donner *et al.* 2003, Klar and Donner 2001, Underwood *et al.* 1998.

2 There has been special interest in recent years in a number of types of PCTs. First, the trials conducted in developing nations to assess whether a limited use of Zidovudine in pregnant women could reduce the rate of transmission of HIV from mother to child have been heavily debated in both the professional literature and popular press. For further discussion of these trials, see Angell (1997), Lurie and Wolf (1997), Phanuphak (1998), Resnik (1998, 2004), Varmus and Satcher (1997). Second, there has been increasing attention to the use of sham surgeries to assess the efficacy of various surgical interventions, including the use of arthroscopic knee surgery to treat osteoarthritis (Moseley *et al.* 2002). For further discussion of sham surgeries, see London and Kadane (2002), Tenery *et al.* (2002).

3 The word "attempt" is used to emphasize that although the obligation of beneficence is often characterized as an obligation to act in the best interests of patients, there are constraints that sometimes make it inappropriate or impossible to do so. These include patients' refusal of consent to treatment, resource limitations, and conflicts among the interests and needs of patients.

4 Therapeutic misconception refers to a phenomenon identified by Appelbaum *et al.* (1982) and confirmed by others whereby research subjects misunderstand the purpose of research and think that research is either an extension of routine care or offers them better treatment. In randomized controlled trials they may think that their physician would ensure that they were given whichever drug he thought was best for them. In PCTs, they think that they will definitely receive the study drug. In phase 1 cancer trials, they think that participation in research offers them a chance for a cure, or for a longer life, or for a better quality of life (Daugherty *et al.* 2000; Yoder *et al.* 1997). For further discussion of the therapeutic misconception, see Dresser 2002.

5 RCTs are not the first avenue for testing new interventions. By the time an RCT is proposed, studies to establish whether there is preliminary evidence of safety and efficacy are conducted to determine whether RCTs are warranted (Levine 1981).

6 One study found that the public favors a relatively even state of disagreement as a necessary condition for permitting RCTs (Johnson *et al.* 1991).

7 An example of the circumstances leading to these scenarios and the consequences is evident in Taylor, Margolese, and Soskolne's (1984) study of surgical principal investigators who were part of the National Surgical Adjuvant Project for Breast and Bowel Cancers. Taylor and colleagues found that a significant number of them enrolled no or few breast cancer patients because they felt that doing so conflicted with their obligations as clinicians.

8 Despite the importance we typically attribute to consensus or widespread agreement in the medical community as indicative or constitutive of knowledge, whether we mean physicians in general or experts, we should not forget those cases in which there has been consensus on the appropriateness or superiority of a treatment we later learned was ineffective or resulted in more harm than good. The history of medicine demonstrates that the clinical community sometimes accepts interventions as standard treatments whose effectiveness and/or safety ought to be questioned, for example, exposing premature infants to high concentrations of oxygen that led to blindness (Cohen 1998) and relying on rest and dietary restrictions to treat ulcers that were caused by bacteria and would only be cured with antibiotic therapy left people suffering from ulcers and limiting their lifestyles for years (NIH 1994).

Although an exploration of these issues is beyond the scope of this chapter, these examples direct us to issues in the philosophy of medicine and the philosophy of science. These include the nature of consensus in the medical community, the failure of consensus to signal knowledge in some cases; the standards for knowledge on which we rely; the extent to which there must be disagreement in the medical community to constitute equipoise; and the mechanisms by which community judgments are made. For further discussion of the philosophy of medicine, see Caplan *et al.* (1981), Engelhardt (2000), Engelhardt and Spicker (1975).

9 See Ludwik Fleck (1979) for a discussion of the sociology of medical knowledge.

10 One might consider patient organizations or advocacy groups' appropriate sources for knowledge of patient values, but these groups are not necessarily representative of the interests or beliefs of all patients with a given condition. (For further discussion of patient advocacy groups, see Dresser (2001) and Quigley (2004).)

11 For further discussion of ethical issues in emergency research, see Brody *et al.* (1997), Fish (1999), Gamelgaard (2004), McRae and Weijer (2002).

12 Statistical significance generally refers to a *p* value of 0.05. But as a number of authors have pointed out, this value, though consistently used in medical research, is arbitrarily chosen and there is nothing inherently normative about it. Some have questioned whether statistical significance always should refer to a *p* value of 0.05. For further discussion of these issues, see Salsburg (1985), Upshur (1999, 2001).

13 For further discussion of surrogate endpoints, see Baker and Kramer (2003), Colburn (2000), Ellenberg (2001), Hughes (2002), Wagner (2002).

14 Although different stopping rules or guidelines are followed, there generally is agreement that to stop a trial early requires a *p* value smaller than the typical $p = 0.05$ (Pocock 1992: 236).

15 Psaty *et al.* (1999) discuss the use of surrogate endpoints in the treatment of cardiovascular disease risk factors, such as hypertension and obesity. They suggest that continued reliance on surrogate endpoints may be appropriate because of the advantages they confer, but that the drug approval process might be changed to include mandatory phase 4 trials so that drugs would be evaluated beyond the surrogate endpoints.

In addition to laboratory and animal testing, the research and development of pharmaceutical products usually involves three or four phases of studies on human subjects. Phase 1 trials assess drug safety. Healthy persons are given escalating doses of the study drug to see how the body responds to it and what doses the human body can tolerate. Phase 2 studies are designed to study a drug's efficacy. RCTs often are employed at this phase to study whether the test drug is efficacious compared to either another drug ACT or placebo PCT. Phase 3 studies also typically are RCTs. They are large studies aimed at assessing a study drug's efficacy and side effects. Phase 4 studies are conducted after a drug is Food and Drug Administration (FDA) approved. These studies may compare a drug to one or more of its competitors in terms of efficacy and/or cost-effectiveness. They may also assess a drug's long-term efficacy and side effects.

Bibliography

Angell, M. (1997) "The Ethics of Clinical Research in the Third World," *New England Journal of Medicine*, 337: 847–49.

Appelbaum, P., Roth, L., and Lidz, C. (1982) "The Therapeutic Misconception: Informed Consent in Psychiatric Research," *International Journal of Law and Psychiatry*, 5: 319–29.

Ashcroft, R. (2001) "Responsibilities of Sponsors are Limited in Premature Discontinuation of Trials," *British Medical Journal*, 323: 53.

——(1999) "Equipoise, Knowledge and Ethics in Clinical Research and Practice," *Bioethics*, 13: 314–26.

Baker, S.G. and Kramer, B.S. (2003) "A Perfect Correlate Does Not a Surrogate Make," *BMC Medical Research Methodology*, 3: 16.

Boyd, K. (2001) "Commentary: Early Discontinuation Violates Helsinki Principles," *British Medical Journal*, 322: 603.

Brant, R., Sutherland, L., and Hilsden, R. (1999) "Examining the Minimum Important Differences," *Statistical Medicine*, 18: 2593–603.

Brody, B. (1998) *The Ethics of Biomedical Research*, New York: Oxford University Press.

Brody, B., Katz, J., and Dula, A. (1997) "In Case of Emergency: No Need for Consent," *Hastings Center Report*, 27(1): 7–12.

Burgh, J. (2000) "Where Next with Stem-Cell-Supported High-Dose Therapy for Breast Cancer?," *The Lancet*, 355: 944–45.

Caplan, A., Engelhardt, H.T., Jr, and McCartney, J. (eds) (1981) *The Concepts of Health and Disease*, Reading, MA: Addison-Wesley.

Cohen, P.J. (1998) "The Placebo is Not Dead: Three Historical Vignettes," *IRB*, 20(2–3): 6–8.

Colburn, W. (2000) "Optimizing the Use of Biomarkers, Surrogate Endpoints, and Clinical Endpoints for More Efficient Drug Development," *Journal of Clinical Pharmacology*, 40: 1419–27.

Daugherty, C.K., Banik, D.M., Janish, L., and Ratain, M.J. (2000) "Quantitative Analysis of Ethical Issues in Phase I Trials: A Survey Interview Study of 144 Advanced Cancer Patients," *IRB*, 22(3): 6–13.

Donner, A., Piaggio, G., and Villar, J. (2003) "Meta-Analyses of Cluster Randomization Trials: Power Considerations," *Evaluation & the Health Professions*, 26: 340–51.

Dresser, R. (2002) "The Ubiquity and Utility of the Therapeutic Misconception," *Social Philosophy and Policy*, 19(2): 271–94.

—— (2001) *When Science Offers Salvation: Patient Advocacy and Research Ethics*, New York: Oxford University Press.

Ellenberg, S. (2001) "Surrogate Endpoints: The Debate Goes On," *Pharmacoepidemiology and Drug Safety*, 10: 493–96.

Emanuel, E. and Miller, F. (2001). "The Ethics of Placebo-Controlled Trials—A Middle Ground," *New England Journal of Medicine*, 345(12): 915–19.

Engelhardt, H.T., Jr (ed.) (2000) *The Philosophy of Medicine: Framing the Field*, Dordrecht: Kluwer Academic Publishers.

Engelhardt, H.T., Jr and Spicker, S.F. (eds) (1975) *Philosophy and Medicine: Evaluation and Explanation in the Biomedical Sciences*, Dordrecht: Reidel.

Evans, S. and Pocock, S. (2001) "Societal Responsibilities of Clinical Trial Sponsors," *British Medical Journal*, 322: 569–70.

Fish, S.S. (1999) "Research Ethics in Emergency Medicine," *Emergency Medicine Clinics of North America*, 17(2): 461–74.

Fisher, L. (1999) "Advances in Clinical Trials in the Twentieth Century," *Annual Review of Public Health*, 20: 109–24.

Fleck, L. (1979) *Genesis and Development of a Scientific Fact*, Chicago, IL: University of Chicago Press.

Freedman, B. (1987) "Equipoise and the Ethics of Clinical Research," *New England Journal of Medicine*, 317: 141–45

Freedman, B., Glass, N., and Weijer, C. (1996a) "Placebo Orthodoxy in Clinical Research. I: Empirical and Methodological Myths," *Journal of Law, Medicine, and Ethics*, 24: 243–51.

—— (1996b) "Placebo Orthodoxy in Clinical Research. II. Ethical, Legal, and Regulatory Myths," *Journal of Law, Medicine, and Ethics*, 24: 252–59.

Fried, C. (1974) *Medical Experimentation: Personal Integrity and Social Policy*, New York: American Elsevier.

Gamelgaard, A. (2004) "Informed Consent in Acute Myocardial Infarction Research," *Journal of Medicine and Philosophy*, 29(4): 417–34.

Giesen, D. (1995) "Civil Liability of Physicians for New Methods of Treatment or Experimentation," *Medical Law Review*, 3: 22–52.

Gifford, F. (1995) "Community-Equipoise and the Ethics of Randomized Clinical Trials," *Bioethics*, 9(2): 127–48.

Glass, N. and Waring, D. (2002) "Effective Trial Design Need Not Conflict with Good Patient Care," *American Journal of Bioethics*, 2(2): 25–26.

Hart, C. (1999) "The Mysterious Placebo Effect," *Modern Drug Discovery*, 2(4): 30–34.

Hellman, D. (2002) "Evidence, Belief, and Action: The Failure of Equipoise to Resolve the Ethical Tension in the Randomized Clinical Trial," *Journal of Law, Medicine, and Ethics*, 30: 375–80.

Hughes, M. (2002) "Evaluating Surrogate Endpoints," *Controlled Clinical Trial*, 23: 703–07.

Iltis, A. (2004) "Placebo Controlled Trials: Restrictions, not Prohibitions," *Cambridge Quarterly of Healthcare Ethics*, 13(4): 380–93.

Johnson, N., Lilford, R.J., and Brazier, W. (1991) "At What Level of Collective Equipoise Does a Clinical Trial Become Ethical?," *Journal of Medical Ethics*, 17: 30–34.

Karlawish, J. and Lantos, J. (1997) "Community Equipoise and the Architecture of Clinical Research," *Cambridge Quarterly of Healthcare Ethics*, 6: 385–96.

Klar, N. and Donner, A. (2001) "Current and Future Challenges in the Design and Analysis of Cluster Randomization Trials," *Statistics in Medicine*, 20: 3729–40.

Kodish, E., Lantos, J., and Siegler, M. (1991) "The Ethics of Randomization," *CA: A Cancer Journal for Clinicians*, 41(3): 180–86.

Lemmens, T. and Miller, P.B. (2002) "Avoiding a Jekyll-Hyde Approach to the Ethics of Clinical Research and Practice," *American Journal of Bioethics*, 2(2):14–17.

Levine, R. (1986) *Ethics and the Regulation of Clinical Research*, 2nd edn, Baltimore: Urban and Schwarzenberg.

——(1985) "The Use of Placebos in Randomized Clinical Trials," *IRB: Review of Human Subjects Research*, 7(2): 1–4.

——(1981) *Ethics and the Regulation of Clinical Research*, Baltimore: Urban and Schwarzenberg.

Lièvre, M.E.B., Menard, J., Bruckert, E., Cogneau, J., Delahaye, F., Giral, P., Leitersdorf, E., Luc, G., Masana, L., Moulin, P., Passa, P., Pouchain, D., and Siest, G. (2001) "Premature Discontinuation of Clinical Trial for Reasons not Related to Efficacy, Safety, or Feasibility," *British Medical Journal*, 322: 603–06.

London, A. and Kadane, J. (2002) "Placebos that Harm: Sham Surgery Controls in Clinical Trials," *Statistical Methods in Medical Research*, 11: 413–27.

Lurie, P. and Wolf, S. (1997) "Unethical Trials of Interventions to Reduce Perinatal Transmission of the HIV in Developing Countries," *New England Journal of Medicine*, 835–56.

McRae, A.D. and Weijer, D. (2002) "Lessons from Everyday Lives: A Moral Justification for Acute Care Research," *Critical Care Medicine*, 30(5): 1146–51.

Miller, F. and Brody, H. (2003) "A Critique of Clinical Equipoise: Therapeutic Misconception in the Ethics of Clinical Trials," *Hastings Center Report*, 33(3): 19–28.

——(2002) "What Makes Placebo-Controlled Trials Unethical?," *American Journal of Bioethics*, 2(2): 3–9.

Moseley, J.B., O'Malley, K., Petersen, N.J., Menke, T.J., Brody, B.A., Kuykendall, D.H., Hollingsworth, J.C., Ashton, C.M., and Wray, N.P. (2002) "A Controlled Trial of Arthroscopic Surgery for Osteoarthritis of the Knee," *New England Journal of Medicine*, 247(2): 81–88.

NIH (1994) "*Helicobacter pylori* in Peptic Ulcer Disease," *NIH Consensus Statement*, 12(1): 1–23.

Phanuphak, P. (1998) "Ethical Issues in Studies in Thailand of the Vertical Transmission of HIV," *New England Journal of Medicine*, 338(12): 834–35.

Pocock, S. (1992) "When to Stop a Clinical Trial," *British Medical Journal*, 305: 235–40.

Podick, D. (1982) "The Randomized Controlled Clinical Trial: Scientific and Ethical Bases," *American Journal of Medicine*, 73: 420–25.

Psaty, B. and Rennie, D. (2003) "Stopping Medical Research to Save Money," *Journal of the American Medical Association*, 289: 2128–31.

Psaty, B.M., Weiss, N.S., Furberg, C.D., Koepsell, T.D., Siscovick, D.S., Rosendaal, F.R., Smith, N.L., Heckbert, S.R., Kaplan, R.C., Lin, D., Fleming, T.R., and Wagner, E.H. (1999) "Surrogate End Points, Health Outcomes, and the Drug-Approval Process for the Treatment of Risk Factors for Cardiovascular Disease," *Journal of the American Medical Association*, 28(8): 786–90.

Quigley, R.B. (2004) "Advocacy and Community: Conflicts of Interest in Public Health Research," in M. Boylan (ed.) *Public Health Policy and Ethics*. New York: Springer.

Resnik, D. (2004) "Biomedical Research in the Developing World: Ethical Issues and Dilemmas," in A. Iltis (ed.) *Research Ethics*. London: Routledge.

——(1998) "The Ethics of HIV Research in Developing Nations," *Bioethics*, 12(4): 286–306.

Rothman, K. and Michels, K. (1994) "The Continuing Unethical Use of Placebo Controls," *New England Journal of Medicine*, 331: 394–98.

Royall, R. (1997) *Statistical Evidence: A Likelihood Paradigm*, London: Chapman and Hall.

Salsburg, D. (1985) "The Religion of Statistics as Practised in Medical Journals," *The American Statistician*, 39: 220–23.

Taylor, K., Margolese, R., and Soskolne, C. (1984) "Physicians' Reasons for not Entering Eligible Patients in a Randomized Clinical Trial of Surgery for Breast Cancer," *The New England Journal of Medicine*, 310: 1363–67.

Temple, R. and Ellenberg, S. (2000a) "Placebo-Controlled Trials and Active-Controlled Trials in the Evaluation of New Treatments: Part 1: Ethical and Scientific Issues," *Annals of Internal Medicine*, 133: 455–63.

——(2000b) "Placebo-Controlled Trials and Active-Controlled Trials in the Evaluation of New Treatments: Part 2: Practical Issues and Specific Cases," *Annals of Internal Medicine*, 133: 464–70.

Tenery, R., Rakatansky, H., Riddick, F.A. Jr, Goldrich, M.S., Morse, L.J., O'Bannon, J.M. 3rd., Ray, P., Smalley, S., Weiss, M., Kao, A., Morin, K., Maixner, A., and Seiden, S. (2002) "Surgical 'Placebo' Controls," *Annals of Surgery*, 235(2): 303–07.

Underwood, M., Barnett, A., and Hajioff, S. (1998) "Cluster Randomization: A Trap for the Unwary," *British Journal of General Practice*, 48(428): 1089–90.

Upshur, R. (2001) "The Ethics of Alpha: Reflections on Statistics Evidence and Values in Medicine," *Theoretical Medicine & Bioethics*, 22: 565–76.

——(1999) "Priors and Prejudice," *Theoretical Medicine & Bioethics*, 20: 319–27.

Varmus, H. and Satcher, D. (1997) "Ethical Complexities of Conducting Research in Developing Countries," *New England Journal of Medicine*, 337(14) :1003–05.

Veatch, R. (2002a) "Subject Indifference and the Justification of Placebo-Controlled Trials," *American Journal of Bioethics*, 2(2): 12–13.

——(2002b) "Indifference of Subjects: An Alternative to Equipoise in Randomized Clinical Trials," *Social Philosophy and Policy*, 19(2): 295–323.

Viberti, G., Slama, G., Pozza, G., Czyzyk, A., Bilous, R.W., Gries, A., Keen, H., Fuller, J.H., and Menzinger, G. (1997) "Early Closure of European Pimagedine Trial," *The Lancet*, 350: 214–15.

Wagner, J. (2002) "Overview of Biomarkers and Surrogate Endpoints in Drug Development," *Disease Markers*, 18: 41–46.

World Medical Association (WMA) (2002) "Declaration of Helsinki Amendment," Online available: http://www.wma.net/e/policy/b3.htm (accessed November 18, 2004).

——(2000) "Declaration of Helsinki: Ethical Principles for Medical Research Involving Human Subjects," *Journal of the American Medical Association*, 284: 3043–45.

Yoder, L.H., O'Rourke, T.J., Etnyre, A., Spears, D.T., and Brown, T.D. (1997) "Expectations and Experiences of Patients with Cancer Participating in Phase I Clinical Trials," *Oncology Nursing Forum*, 24: 891–96.

6   Ethics in behavioral and social science research

James M. DuBois

Nietzsche wrote, "What does not kill me makes me stronger." But not everyone is dismissive of harms lesser than death, just as not everyone wrests benefits from trials and tribulations. This, in short, explains why we are concerned with ethics in behavioral and social science (BSS) research. BSS research is unlikely to kill anyone, but some of it presents harms that are not insignificant and much of it fails to make us stronger. What follows is a survey of the most common ethical issues that are faced in BSS research along with procedural recommendations that can assist researchers in addressing these issues.

Two focal examples of BSS research

As we consider benefits, risks, privacy concerns, and informed consent in BSS research, it will be helpful to have two clear examples of BSS research in mind that together illustrate most of the issues that will be visited.

The Tearoom Trade *study*

From 1965 to 1968 Laud Humphreys conducted dissertation research on men who have impersonal sex with men (Humphreys 1970). Without disclosing his role as a sociology researcher, Humphreys played the role of "watch queen," that is, he looked out for intruders while men performed oral sex on men in the public restrooms of a St Louis park. He later disclosed his role to some men he had observed and interviewed them on their daily lives. In other cases, he recorded his subjects' license plate numbers to track where they lived. A year later, after changing his hair and attire, he interviewed these same men in their homes under the guise of conducting an anonymous public health survey. Among the positive outcomes Humphreys cites was dispelling myths that the men he studied are dangerous homosexual deviants: he found that most were married to women and had children; only 14 percent were exclusively homosexual and identified themselves as gay. Many within the gay community welcomed his research and in some police districts it lead to decreased raids and sodomy arrests.

The Profiles of Student Life *studies*

Over 1 million students in the United States have participated in studies using the *Search Institute Profiles of Student Life: Attitudes and Behavior* (Profiles) survey (Search Institute 2001). Far from being a dramatic classic case of research like the Tearoom Trade study or Milgram's obedience studies (Milgram 1974), these studies have been conducted in over 1,000 communities since 1989 and continue today. They often bring together BSS researchers from education, public health, and developmental psychology. Not only does the 156-item Profiles survey assess developmental assets like positive relationships, opportunities, skills, and values, but it also assesses deficits like being overexposed to television, being left at home alone, and being physically abused, as well as high-risk behavior patterns and traits such as illegal drug use, sexual intercourse, depression, and attempted suicide. It is typically administered in schools to students in sixth through twelfth grade. The Search Institute claims that results of the survey can enhance "asset-building opportunities" in many parts of local communities, including youth-serving organizations, parent groups, law enforcement, and congregations.

What constitutes BSS research?

What separates BSS studies like the Tearoom Trade study or the Profiles survey studies from biomedical research? While this question may seem purely academic, it takes on practical importance as society wrestles with whether and how BSS research should be subjected to ethical review. BSS researchers have long protested that the standards used to review biomedical research are not appropriate for BSS research; they may do little to foster human protections, and may unnecessarily slow or prevent the conduct of research (Azar 2002; Douglas 1979; Pattullo 1982). Yet the boundaries between, say, biomedical research and BSS research are often vague. Consider the broad spectrum of studies that might be conducted to improve understanding of drug addiction behavior:

- a survey of high school students that examines the correlation between self-reported drug abuse and developmental assets;
- an ethnographic study in which a researcher lives on the streets with drug addicts to observe how people obtain illegal narcotics, how they obtain the needed money, and how frequently they use drugs;
- an epidemiological study using medical records to determine whether mental health diagnoses like depression are correlated with addictive behavior;
- an experimental test of the relative efficacy of two addiction-counseling techniques;
- a study that collects blood samples from addicted and non-addicted people to determine genetic correlates to addiction;
- a study that administers narcotics to people who are actively abusing drugs to determine the brain mechanisms that are activated by narcotics and may play a role in addiction.

All of these studies are focused on addictive behavior, yet they range from those we intuitively label as BSS to those we label as biomedical. One way of describing the difference is to define BSS research as research that studies behavioral and social variables without an involuntary biological independent variable (in which case only the last two studies would count as biomedical). But perhaps it is simplest and most honest to acknowledge that labeling BSS research is a matter of convention that is per se of little importance. What is more important is determining (a) whether a study actually constitutes research, (b) the kinds and levels of risk a study poses, and (c) the competencies that institutional review board (IRB) or other reviewers need to provide ethical review. Ethical issues are only rarely affected by whether the researchers belong to the field of anthropology, economics, health services, medicine, public health, psychology, or sociology, or whether the IRB providing review is labeled biomedical or BSS.[1]

What constitutes research?

The question whether a study actually constitutes research is frequently raised in BSS fields. US regulations define research as "a systematic investigation, including research development, testing and evaluation, designed to develop or contribute to generalizable knowledge" (45CFR46.102.d). BSS educators frequently conduct classroom "research projects" with human participants strictly for educational purposes without intending to contribute to generalizable knowledge. Regardless of risks to participants, these are typically not treated as research unless students or professors intend to publish or publicly disseminate results (as this supposedly betrays an intention to contribute to generalizable knowledge).

Quality assessment and services studies likewise may be systematic and may use common BSS research tools like valid, randomly distributed questionnaires, but they do not typically count as research unless there is an accompanying intention to publicly share generalizable knowledge. For example, using the Profiles survey might not count as research if the only purpose is to profile a local population for the purpose of shaping student services. However, even when such studies will be shared publicly, their ethical review may still diverge from the typical review of research, especially with regard to informed consent. Because educators or service providers may have legitimate claims to *gathering* data without informed consent for non-research purposes (e.g., student assessment or improved care of one's patients), it is sometimes appropriate to seek informed consent only for the *public use* of data (DuBois 2002). However, building a partnership with participants through the informed consent process may improve the quality (e.g., sincerity) of data gathered, even if participation rates may decrease.

Perhaps the most difficult cases to decide involve qualitative studies. It is sometimes said that qualitative studies by nature do not contribute to generalizable knowledge, but rather focus on individual cases in order to provide insight and understanding that may or may not be used to generate hypotheses and theories. Regardless whether one believes that the outcomes of qualitative research contribute to the development of generalizable knowledge, the trend is to treat qualitative studies as research when an intention exists to publish or otherwise publicly share findings. While this makes sense insofar as there are human participants and some level of risk exists, it is often difficult to find principled distinctions between many of the BSS projects that we treat as research and other activities such as journalism, medical case reports, and government-mandated educational tests whose results are publicly disseminated (Pritchard 2001).

Value in BSS research and its ethical review

Once it is determined that a study counts as research, the first significant ethical question is whether it offers value sufficient to justify participation. We saw that both the Tearoom Trade study and the Profiles survey claim to offer the benefit of new knowledge that is useful for members of the populations studied; in the one case by reducing stigma, in the other by empowering those who serve students. Both, however, also illustrate that determination of value can be controversial: some might not consider decreased raids on so-called tearooms a desirable outcome, and others might find statistics on local teenage drug use stigmatizing.

The value that research offers to participants and communities may be as varied as the basic needs that human beings have. For example, benefits may include knowledge, skills, valuable relationships with researchers and agencies, empowerment, material resources, and improved clinical therapies (Sieber 1992). However, studies that fail to offer any value whatsoever are by nature unethical as they fail any conceivable benefit-burden test. They are not considered merely neutral in value because at the least they waste time and resources; they may also undermine trust in research and willingness to participate in research in the future.

Value and scientific merit

While many researchers resist the idea that scientific review should be part of the ethical review of research, some minimal consideration of design and power are appropriate insofar as invalid or unreliable research *cannot* offer value (Freedman 1987). However, given the plurality of scientific worldviews—especially within BSS fields (just think of the wars between quantitatively and qualitatively minded researchers)— reviewers should exercise considerable caution when evaluating scientific merit and should disapprove studies only when they commit what are commonly recognized to be egregious violations of scientific standards for gaining new knowledge.

Risks in BSS research

Risk assessment in research involves attempting to identify the (1) kinds, (2) magnitude, (3) probability of harm a study presents, as well as (4) the stakeholders who might be affected by a harm. While this sometimes involves little more than an exercise of the imagination, several thoughtful frameworks exist for addressing the various kinds of harms that can arise in BSS research (Koocher 2002; Sieber 1992; Warwick 1982).

Forms of harm

The major forms of harm that threaten participants are listed in *The Belmont Report* (National Commission 1979):

1. Psychological: e.g., boredom, anxiety, embarrassment, or psychotic relapse;
2. Physical: e.g., sexual dysfunction, high blood pressure, or suicide;
3. Legal: e.g., fines or imprisonment;
4. Social: e.g., stigmatization, harm to reputation, or divorce;
5. Economic: lost time at work, loss of employment, legal fees or medical bills for harms incurred in research.

Moving beyond this generic consideration of harms to a more specific assessment of risks requires consideration of the study design used and the populations from which participants will be drawn.

Risk and study designs

Assessing risk obviously requires consideration of specific details of a study's design. However, a review of the literature shows that certain methodologies raise certain kinds of concerns more frequently than others. Table 6.1 presents an overview of several BSS methodologies and the main risks that are commonly identified in the literature.

Special populations and kinds of vulnerability

BSS research is frequently conducted with populations that may generate special ethical issues. Special populations include students (DuBois 2002; Fisher 2003; Koocher and Keith-Spiegel 1998); children (Grisso 1992; Hoagwood *et al.* 1996; Koocher and Keith-Spiegel 1990); elderly people (Lane *et al.* 1990; Russell 1999); prisoners (Jenkins-Hall and Osborn 1994; Mastroianni and Kahn 2001); people with cognitive disorders (Annas and Glantz 1997; Appelbaum *et al.* 1999; NBAC 1999); and people with human immunodeficiency virus (HIV)/acquired immunodeficiency syndrome (AIDS) (Committee for the Protection 1986; Sieber and Sorensen 1992).

Regulations have been created to protect some special populations, for example, prisoners and children (US 45CFR46, subparts C and D, respectively). However, the National Bioethics Advisory Committee (NBAC) has recently recommended an approach that focuses on the kinds of vulnerability rather than on special populations (2001). Kinds of vulnerability include cognitive or communicative vulnerability, deferential vulnerability, medical vulnerability, economic vulnerability, and social vulnerability. Each one of these vulnerabilities refers to an increase in one or more risk (sometimes the magnitude, but typically the probability of a harm). For example, cognitive or communicative vulnerability may heighten the risk that a participant is insufficiently able to comprehend information, deliberate, and make or express decisions, which increases the likelihood that informed consent will not be properly obtained and participants will be less able to protect their interests. Each of the six vulnerabilities calls for special safeguards, although these need to be tailored to

Table 6.1 Common risks of BSS methodologies

Methodology	Special risks[a]	Literature
BSS research in general	Loss of confidentiality with attending risks (e.g., economic, legal, social); confidentiality may restrict ability to intervene, report, or assist as needed; results may stigmatize groups; consent may be compromised or absent; embarrassment or discomfort; lost time and inconvenience	(Beauchamp *et al.* 1982; Boruch and Cecil 1983; Kelman 1982; Sieber 1992; Sieber and Stanley 1998)
Qualitative interviews	Loss of confidentiality due to recording and level of biographical detail; disclosure of details about third parties; response bias (e.g., desire to please interviewer); unstructured designs make informed consent difficult	(Gallant 2002; Hadjistavropoulos and Smythe 2001; Shaw 2003; Smythe and Murray 2000)
Focus groups	Loss of confidentiality due to disclosure in group setting and recording methods; disclosure of details about third party; response bias (e.g., group think, desire to please interviewer)	(Gallant 2002; Smith 1995)
Questionnaires/ written surveys	Loss of confidentiality if written record is not protected; consent is often passive or implied; closed items may reduce control over disclosure	(Evans *et al.* 2002; Oakes 2002)
Observation/ ethnography	When overt: discomfort; loss of privacy. When covert: no consent; privacy intrusion; no control over disclosure	(Marshall 1992; Parrot 2002; Shaw 2003)
Record review/ existing data review	Loss of confidentiality if data is not sufficiently de-identified or protected; consent is often waived thereby decreasing control over access	(Speer 2002; Steinberg 1983)
Experimental designs	Known effective intervention may be withheld; interferes with individualizing treatment or intervention; participants typically are unaware of group assignment	(FDA 1999; Freedman 1990; Koocher 2002; Oakley 1998)

Note

a The term "special risks" does not imply that they are exclusive to the method, but rather that the method has features that heighten such risks. General risks that run equally across methods are not repeated for each method (e.g., stigma or harms resulting from loss of confidentiality), nor are variations on methods addressed (e.g., use of deception in ethnography).

the specific study and the specific heightened risks. For example, participants with cognitive vulnerability may need an assessment of decision-making capacity and their wishes or interests may need to be protected using advanced directives or surrogate decision-makers (Berg and Appelbaum 1999).

This approach to vulnerability has clear advantages. As NBAC noted, regulations may become unnecessarily unwieldy if we seek to craft special regulations for each vulnerable group: many different groups require the same kinds of protections; the status of groups changes with time; some individuals may belong to more than one vulnerable group, and different members of groups may have different needs and vulnerabilities (2001).

Nevertheless, focusing on individual participants may not be possible for review boards and members of local communities may indeed share special needs. Moreover, many of the same kinds of risks that threaten individuals may also threaten communities. For example, when the results of poorly conducted research or research on sensitive and stigmatizing issues find their way into peer-reviewed literature and eventually into public media, they can contribute to widespread poor health practices, stigmatization of groups, wasted research and health dollars, and mental anguish among those affected by these harms (Levine 1988). Thus, a shift in focus from vulnerable groups to kinds of vulnerability in no way diminishes the need for or benefits of community consultation in the design and development of research (CDC *et al.* 1998; Fisher and Wallace 2000).

Protecting privacy

Privacy violations in BSS research can lead to every one of the harms identified in *The Belmont Report*. For example, although Humphreys does not report any breaches of confidentiality in the Tearoom Trade study, public disclosure that a married man had paid for oral sex in a tearoom might cause psychological harms (embarrassment and anxiety), economic harms (loss of employment), social harms (divorce or loss of friends), and possibly even physical harm (from angry spouses or "gay bashers"). Because the risks attending to privacy violations are among the most common and significant in BSS research, matters of privacy and confidentiality deserve special attention. After clarifying basic terms, the two focal examples of research presented above will be used to illustrate the major issues that arise in protecting the privacy of individuals and the confidentiality of their research data.

Key definitions

Drawing from the work of Boruch and Cecil (1979) and Seiber (2001a) we may define privacy as "the interest people have in controlling the access of others to themselves." Confidentiality may be defined as "agreements about how identifiable information will be handled to protect the interest people have in controlling access to themselves." These agreements may be explicit (e.g., written) or implied by society's understanding of the role one is playing in relationship to others (e.g., priest, therapist, or researcher). Ethical agreements may extend beyond legal agreements and vice versa. Information may include oral or written information, audio recordings, or stored images of or about an individual. Identifiers include anything that links information to a specific individual either by itself (e.g., names, social security numbers, photographs) or taken together with other information (e.g., a combination of age, race, and place of employment). Using the definition of confidentiality offered above, we understand that de-identified data is not confidential as it cannot be linked to an individual. However, the related term "anonymous" is frequently used much too loosely; the absence of a name on a form or recording does not automatically entail that the collective information it contains cannot be used to identify an individual.[2] For this reason, the more precise term "de-identified" is preferable to the term "anonymous."

Privacy as distinct from confidentiality

The Tearoom Trade study exquisitely illustrates privacy concerns as distinct from confidentiality concerns. While Humphreys tells readers that he protected the confidentiality of the data he gathered, his methodology deprived his subjects of the opportunity to control his access to them *as a researcher*. We allow different people different degrees of access to ourselves; what we feel comfortable telling a therapist or spouse we may not feel comfortable telling a reporter, employer, or researcher. Presumably, his subjects gave him access to observe their behavior in his role of "watch queen" but most would have denied him that access as researcher. In any case, we do not know how they would have responded because he did not obtain informed consent, which is the normal mechanism used to enable people to exercise control over the access researchers have to them in the context of research.

The degree of a given privacy violation depends on both the kind of behavior (whether it is generally regarded as private, like sex, or public, like driving) and the setting (whether it is generally regarded as private, like a bedroom, or public, like a highway). Covert research on public behaviors in public settings is generally considered acceptable; covert research on private behavior in private settings is generally forbidden; other forms of covert research tend to generate the bulk of controversy. Additionally, determining which behaviors and places are regarded as private is no easy task given developmental and cultural variations in views toward privacy (Laufer and Wolfe 1977; Sieber 2001a). For this reason, community consultation is often essential to determining what privacy protections should be put in place.

Privacy, confidentiality, and existing data

Another common form of research combines concerns about privacy and confidentiality, namely, research using existing data. For example, the Search Institute keeps and uses all data gathered from local schools using the Profiles survey (2001). Insofar as data is identifiable, this raises a matter of privacy because individuals may not have granted consent to third parties to use their data. Current US regulations require that if consent has not been granted for the use of existing data, then data must be de-identified prior to use (Barnes and Gallin 2003). Insofar as permission is granted, the data must be still treated confidentially.

Confidentiality across the life of a study

Even if one plans to publish only de-identified and aggregated data, if data is identifiable in the form it is gathered, it must be treated as confidential and protections should be put in place across the life of the study. Any limitations to one's ability to protect the confidentiality of data (e.g., compliance with mandatory reporting laws) should be disclosed to participants during the informed consent process (Appelbaum and Rosenbaum 1989; Haggerty and Hawkins 2000). Table 6.2 presents common strategies for protecting confidentiality at different stages and in different forms of research.

The National Institutes of Health (NIH) provides researchers with Certificates of Confidentiality (COCs) for research that gathers identifiable information that could have adverse consequences for participants, including legal risks or damage to their financial standing, employability, insurability, and reputation. Researchers do not need to be funded by the NIH in order to apply for a COC. COCs allow the investigator and others who have access to research records to refuse to disclose identifying information on research participants in any civil, criminal, administrative, legislative, or other proceeding, whether at the federal, state, or local level (2004). A COC does not protect participants from *voluntary* disclosure of information by the investigator, for example, if the investigator complies with state laws mandating the report of child abuse. However, investigators are obliged to disclose in the informed consent process any conditions under which confidentiality will be breached.

Informed consent

As noted earlier, informed consent is the ordinary mechanism used to enable participants to control access of others to themselves. It is considered as not only an exercise of autonomy or self-determination (Beauchamp and Childress 2001), but also an important form of self-protection and accordingly a means of respecting the principle of nonmaleficence. *The Belmont Report* presents commonly recognized requirements of valid informed consent: presenting all information that a "reasonable volunteer" would consider material to deciding whether to participate in a study; presenting this information in a manner that is understandable; ascertaining that the potential participant has understood the information; and providing conditions for consent that are free of coercion or undue influence (National Commission 1979).

The Nuremberg Code, which was developed following the abuse of subjects by Nazi researchers, treats informed consent as an ethical imperative. Its first line reads, "The voluntary consent of the human subject is absolutely essential" (Annas and Grodin 1992: 2). Yet the Nuremberg Code addressed medical experimentation; its authors apparently did not have in mind BSS research, which often challenges the feasibility and the ethical imperative of obtaining valid informed consent.

What follows is an outline of several current ethical dilemmas that face BSS researchers as they balance the aims of respecting the self-determination of participants with generating valid, reliable, and useful knowledge.

Table 6.2 Examples of confidentiality protection at different phases of research

Research phase	Confidentiality protection	Useful literature
Prior to beginning research	• Consider whether a COC[a] is needed to prevent the subpoena of research data • Obtain consent as appropriate • Identify a complaint mechanism for participants	(Hoagwood 1994; Kelsey 1981; Wolf *et al.* 2004)
Conducting interviews	• Provide a private setting • Train interpreters, facilitators, and other participants to respect confidentiality • Discourage use of names when referring to self and third parties	(Sieber 2001b; Smith 1995; Tangney 2000)
Obtaining existing data from a database	• Remove identifiers using "safe harbor" or statistical criteria • Use as few identifying variables as possible; remove when no longer needed	(Barnes and Gallin 2003; Kelsey 1981; Simon *et al.* 2000; Steinberg 1983; Wallace Jr 1982)
Surveys or research requiring recontacting or data linking	• Link data to codes or aliases • Eliminate need to store code sheet by allowing participants to memorize or store code in sealed envelope • Explore alternative linking systems	(Black and Hodge 1987; Boruch 1982; Boruch and Cecil 1979; Sieber 2001a)
Data storage	• Data stored using codes if re-identification or linking is needed • Code sheets kept separately with restricted access • Restrict paper access using two locks (office, file cabinet) • Restrict electronic access using firewalls, unique passwords, audit trails, and other technology as appropriate given risks and resources	(Fisher 2003; Health Privacy Working Group 1999; National Research Council 1997; Rada 2003)
Data analysis and presentation	• Use only as many variables as needed • Use only aggregated data or else remove identifiers in narratives • Use statistical analysis or safe harbor techniques to ensure de-identification	(Boruch 1982; Boruch and Cecil 1979; National Library of Medicine 1996; Rada 2003)
Data destruction	• Finely shred paper and properly dispose • Degauss (demagnetize) tapes • Consult with information technology personnel to permanently delete electronic data and destroy removable data storage systems	(Rada 2003; Saint Louis University 2004)

Note
a COC refers to Certificate of Confidentiality.

Consent versus assent

Ordinarily minors are not allowed to give informed consent; however, once old enough, they should be asked to assent to participation in research and their parents or legal guardians should be asked to grant permission (Koocher and Keith-Spiegel 1990). Should parental permission ever be waived for research involving children or adolescents? For example, should the assent of a 14 year old suffice for participation in a smoking cessation study when teenagers are unwilling to let their parents know they smoke (Grisso 1992; Sieber 1992)? Should a child ever be included in research without assent (Koocher and Keith-Spiegel 1990), for example, when an experimental treatment appears promising?

Passive and implied consent

The concept of implied consent has a limited place in research that is either exempt or in which consent has been waived. It is commonly cited as the form of permission obtained in survey research, for example, when a person returns a mailed survey. Implied consent rests on the fairly reasonable assumption that people who do not wish to participate in a survey will make this known by not participating; in contrast, those who complete and return surveys agree to participate. However, implied consent still requires that participants be adequately informed (e.g., in a cover letter) and that it be made clear that participation is voluntary.

So-called passive consent is more controversial and is typically used with parents whose children are potential participants. Passive consent involves only informing the parent about a study and providing information on how to opt out; by default, the child becomes a participant. (This, for example, is the form of consent that the Search Institute generally recommends when the Profiles survey is used.) However, passive consent runs the risk of being no consent whatsoever; from the absence of a response one cannot infer that a parent has received, read, and understood information mailed to an address, nor that they have agreed to their child's participation (Hoagwood *et al.* 1996). Thus, it should not really be called a form of consent, and should be reserved only for studies that are ethically deemed to meet the criteria for a waiver of consent (45CFR46.116.c).

Third party and community consent

In the course of focus groups or interviews, participants may divulge information about others (e.g., parents, sexual partners, employers) that could put these third parties at risk. At what point is it appropriate to treat third parties as participants, and how feasible is obtaining consent without violating the privacy of persons interviewed? The National Research Council has suggested that "no hard-and-fast rules can or should apply," but decisions must take into account the specifics of a study including risks, setting, the nature of the data gathered, and the characteristics of the study population (1997: 99).

Some qualitative recruiting techniques involve indirect recruitment; for example, so-called snowball sampling involves asking participants to recommend other potential participants who fit a certain profile (e.g., others infected with HIV from intravenous (IV) drug use). While this can be an effective way of recruiting hard-to-reach populations, in effect, it involves asking participants to disclose sensitive details about individuals without their permission. Direct recruitment that uses participants to "advertise" a study often provides a viable alternative. For example, participants may be asked to contact other potential participants and provide them with the researcher's name and contact information (Margolis 2000).

Even when it is feasible to get consent from individual participants, research often affects communities in fairly direct ways, for example, by reinforcing negative stereotypes (CDC *et al.* 1998). Even when individual consent is obtained, some have suggested that communities also should be consulted when research results may negatively impact a community.

Other studies raise the issue of community permission with even greater force. For example, a study that involves observing behavior in school halls or the use of anti-smoking billboards may deprive individuals of the opportunity to opt out. In such cases, some speak of the need to obtain community consent (Weijer 1999). However, Macklin observes that the idea of group consent is problematic given that groups rarely enjoy 100 percent consensus on issues. She cites Shelling, who notes that even if, for pragmatic reasons, a decision whether to conduct a school-based community health project might rest on whether 50 percent or more of parents agree, this "probably should not be referred to as 'consent'" (Macklin 1982: 210). Moreover, some communities do not espouse democratic ideals. In such situations, is the consent of a tribal leader or of the men of a group sufficient to justify the participation of all—including women and children?

While these issues are complex and the language of consent may be inappropriate when groups are subjects, some form of community education, input, and acceptance seems essential to the ethical justification and frequently the feasibility of a study (CDC *et al.* 1998; Sieber 1992).

Deception

Alan Elms has observed that our use of the term "deception" is "so sweeping that it includes Satan's lures for lost souls, the traitor's treachery, the false lover's violation of a pure heart. How could any deception ever be considered ethically justifiable if it keeps such company?" (Elms 1982: 232).

Many forms of deception exist in research (Sieber 1982b); for example, Humphreys' methodology involved both covert research and deception insofar as he led others to believe his main interest was being a watch queen. But Humphreys' research was far from unique insofar as it used deception: some form of deception was used in roughly 50 percent of all studies conducted in social psychology in the 1970s and 1980s (Korn 1997; Sieber *et al.* 1995).

Is it ever right to deny people informed consent to gather identifiable details about them as is done in covert research? Is it ever right to mislead people about the variables a study is investigating or their role in the study?

Humphreys (1970), Milgram (1964), and others (Douglas 1979) have argued that privacy and autonomy rights must be limited by our need for other goods and that some important knowledge cannot be gained without the use of deceptive or covert techniques. Moreover, some surveys have found that a majority of people supports the use of deceptive methods in research when important knowledge can be gained (Lustig *et al.* 1993; Milgram 1974).

In contrast, others have argued that such methods are not only disrespectful and potentially harmful to subjects, but also may undermine trust in researchers, encourage insincere forms of participation, and eventually harm science rather than foster its interest (Baumrind 1964; Sieber 1982b; Warwick 1982).

Professional ethics codes and regulations have typically adopted a middle course, granting discretion to researchers and IRBs to determine whether the use of deceptive methods is justified in specific cases with special protections in place. For example, the American Psychological Association's (APA) code of ethics states:

> (a) Psychologists do not conduct a study involving deception unless they have determined that the use of deceptive techniques is justified by the study's significant prospective scientific, educational, or applied value and that effective nondeceptive alternative procedures are not feasible.
>
> (b) Psychologists do not deceive prospective participants about research that is reasonably expected to cause physical pain or severe emotional distress.
>
> (c) Psychologists explain any deception that is an integral feature of the design and conduct of an experiment to participants as early as is feasible, preferably at the conclusion of their participation, but no later than at the conclusion of the data collection, and permit participants to withdraw their data.
>
> (See also Standard 8.08, Debriefing.) (APA 2002: 8.07)

As the code suggests, the use of deceptive methods is justified—if at all—only after alternative designs have been explored. Several articles suggest designs that may yield trustworthy data in the place of deception designs (Sieber 1992).

Some authors explore forms of consent or permission (e.g., prospective community permission or disclosure that some variables are being covertly investigated) that may be used when deceptive or covert research is conducted (Pittenger 2002; Soble 1978). While these are not always feasible, Elms suggests that the fact that researchers tend to publish the results of studies that use deception allows for a level of transparency and oversight that sets researchers apart from (other) "con artists" (Elms 1982).

As noted earlier, the American Psychological Association (APA) code generally encourages debriefing participants after deception has been used, but the APA code, US regulations, and many ethicists allow the use of discretion when debriefing is expected to be more harmful than beneficial (Hoagwood *et al.* 1996; Sieber 1982a).

Ethics and IRB review of BSS research

BSS researchers have often complained that IRB review unfairly treats BSS research as though it were high-risk biomedical research. This is often blamed on regulations that were supposedly written with biomedical research in mind. However, many nations do not regulate BSS research at all, and US regulations, in fact, grant IRBs tremendous discretion in the review of BSS research. Much of BSS research is exempt from the regulations, leaving IRBs free to establish their own review policies (45CFR46.101.b). Accordingly, IRBs may allow the use of existing data even without consent when no identifiers are used (45CFR46.101.b.4). Under specific conditions informed consent may be waived (45CFR46.116.c); parental permission may be waived (45CFR46.408d); permission to conduct research that involves some element of deception or nondisclosure may be granted; and IRBs may waive the requirement to obtain a signed consent form, for example, when the signed form would pose the only threat to confidentiality (45CFR46.117.c). That is to say, IRBs are given the discretion to approach ethical questions in BSS research precisely as ethical and not merely regulatory or compliance questions.[3] Thus, much of the frustration BSS researchers are experiencing with IRB review processes stems from the modus operandi IRBs have freely adopted rather than with the regulatory framework (De Vries *et al.* 2004).

Moreover, BSS researchers have their own significant role to play in improving the value of ethical review. A growing number of BSS researchers are acknowledging that while normative ethics may provide principles to guide human actions (e.g., autonomy, beneficence, and justice), empirical research is needed to guide us in determining how these principles are best applied (De Vries *et al.* 2004; Stanley and Guido 1996; Stanley *et al.* 1996). For example, autonomy may require us to obtain informed consent, but BSS research may clarify how a variety of factors influence consent, including the readability of forms, cultural factors, cognitive capacities, and age (Stanley and Guido 1996). Likewise, ethicists may speak of the need to protect privacy, but BSS researchers have contributed significantly to our understanding of what protections participants want and to strategies for guaranteeing protection (Boruch and Cecil 1979, 1983). In recent years the NIH, the Office of Research Integrity, and other government agencies have provided funding to support BSS researchers to conduct research on research ethics, thus encouraging and enabling such BSS research.

As BSS researchers engage in dialogue with IRBs and community members to improve the ethical review of research, they must not view their efforts as a distraction from the aims of science. Ethical review can indeed unnecessarily hamper the progress of research, but it can also contribute significantly to the value of BSS research. For example, participants who have doubts about confidentiality may be unwilling to answer questions forthrightly; participants who believe they are being deceived about a study design may treat research like a game; and participants who believe they have benefited from past research will be more willing to participate in research again (Getz and Borfitz 2002; Sieber 1992). In the end, creative problem solving in BSS research can contribute to the respectful treatment of participants and the development of new and generalizable knowledge.

Notes

1 In special circumstances the specific protections that a researcher offers to participants may vary from field to field. For example, in the United States few states require all persons to

report child abuse, but all states require health-care providers (e.g., licensed psychologists) to report. See http://www.smith-lawfirm.com/mandatory_reporting.htm, last visited May 27, 2004. Thus, there may be a legal difference in the extent to which a sociologist versus a psychologist is expected to protect confidentiality. Similarly, given expectations of physicians to provide the best care possible to patients, they may have a heightened duty to clarify what benefits may be reasonably expected and to discuss alternatives to participation (Appelbaum *et al.* 1987).

2 For example, while the Profiles information booklet claims the survey is anonymous—and indeed names are not gathered—it collects sufficient demographic variables to identify some students (e.g., the one female Asian student living with one parent who attends a specific school).

3 As they do so, IRB members and researchers may find it helpful to consult a guidance document prepared by the National Science Foundation which illustrates ways that ethical issues in BSS research can be resolved within the US regulatory framework (NSF 2002).

Bibliography

American Psychological Association (APA) (2002) "Ethical Principles of Psychologists and Code of Conduct," Online available: http://www.apa.org/ethics/code2002.pdf (accessed June 2, 2004).

Annas, G.J. and Glantz, L.H. (1997) "Informed Consent to Research on Institutionalized Mentally Disabled Persons: The Dual Problems of Incapacity and Voluntariness," in A.E. Shamoo (ed.) *Ethics in Neurobiological Research with Human Subjects: The Baltimore Conference on Ethics* (pp. 55–80). Amsterdam: Gordon and Breach Publishers.

Annas, G.J. and Grodin, M.A. (eds) (1992) *The Nazi Doctors and the Nuremberg Code: Human Rights in Human Experimentation*, New York: Oxford University Press.

Appelbaum, P.S. and Rosenbaum, A. (1989) "Tarasoff and the Researcher: Does the Duty to Protect Apply in the Research Setting?," *American Psychologist*, 44(6): 885–94.

Appelbaum, P.S., Dresser, R., Fisher, C.B., Moreno, J.D., and Saks, E.R. (1999) *Research Involving Persons with Mental Disorders that may Affect Decisionmaking Capacity*, Rockville: National Bioethics Advisory Commission.

Appelbaum, P.S., Roth, L.H., Lidz, C.W., Benson, P., and Winslade, W.J. (1987) "False Hopes and Best Data: Consent to Research and the Therapeutic Misconception," *Hastings Center Report*, 17(2): 20–24.

Azar, B. (2002) "Ethics at the Cost of Research?," *Monitor on Psychology*, 33(2): 42.

Barnes, M. and Gallin, K.E. (2003) " 'Exempt' Research after the Privacy Rule," *IRB: Ethics & Human Research*, 25(4): 5–6.

Baumrind, D. (1964) "Some Thoughts on Ethics of Research: After Reading Milgram's 'Behavioral Study of Obedience'," *American Psychologist*, 19: 421–23.

Beauchamp, T.L. and Childress, J.F. (2001) *Principles of Biomedical Ethics*, 5th edn, New York: Oxford University Press.

Beauchamp, T.L., Faden, R.R., Wallace, R.J., and Walters, L. (eds) (1982) *Ethical Issues in Social Science Research*, Baltimore, MD: Johns Hopkins University Press.

Berg, J.W. and Appelbaum, P.S. (1999) "Subjects' Capacity to Consent to Neurobiological Research," in H.A. Pincus, J.A. Lieberman, and S. Ferris (eds) *Ethics in Psychiatric Research: A Resource Manual for Human Subjects Protection* (pp. 81–106). Washington, DC: American Psychiatric Association.

Black, K.J. and Hodge, M.H. (1987) "Protecting Subjects' Identity in Test–Retest Experiments," *IRB: A Review of Human Subjects Research*, 9(2): 10–11.

Boruch, R.F. (1982) "Methods for Resolving Privacy Problems in Social Research," in T.L. Beauchamp, R.R. Faden, R.J. Wallace, and L. Walters (eds) *Ethical Issues in Social Science Research* (pp. 292–314). Baltimore, MD: Johns Hopkins University Press.

Boruch, R.F. and Cecil, J.S. (eds) (1983) *Solutions to Ethical and Legal Problems in Social Research*, New York: Academic Press.

——(1979) *Assuring the Confidentiality of Social Research Data*, Philadelphia, PA: University of Pennsylvania Press.

Centers for Disease Control and Prevention (CDC), Department of Health & Human Services (DHHS), National Institutes of Health (NIH), Food and Drug Administration (FDA), Human Resources and Services Administration, Substance Abuse and Mental Health Services Administration, and Indian Health Service (1998) *Building Community Partnerships in Research: Recommendations and Strategies*, Washington, DC: Government Printing Office.

Committee for the Protection of Human Participants in Research, APA (1986) "Ethical Issues in Psychological Research on AIDS," *IRB: A Review of Human Subjects Research*, 8(4): 8–10.

De Vries, R., DeBruin, D.A., and Goodgame, A. (2004) "Ethics Review of Social, Behavioral, and Economic Research: Where Should We Go from Here?," *Ethics & Behavior*, 14(4): 351–68.

Douglas, J.D. (1979) "Living Morality Versus Bureaucratic Fiat," in C.B. Klockars and F.W. O'Connor (eds) *SAGE Annual Reviews of Studies in Deviance: Vol. 3. Deviance and Decency*, (pp. 13–34). Beverly Hills, CA: Sage Publications.

DuBois, J. (2002) "When Is Informed Consent Appropriate in Educational Research?," *IRB: Ethics & Human Research*, 24(1): 1–8.

Elms, A.C. (1982) "Keeping Deception Honest: Justifying Conditions for Social Scientific Research Stratagems," in T.L. Beauchamp, R.R. Faden, R.J. Wallace, and L. Walters (eds) *Ethical Issues in Social Science Research* (pp. 232–45). Baltimore, MD: Johns Hopkins University Press.

Evans, M., Robling, M., Maggs Rapport, F., Houston, H., Kinnersley, P., and Wilkinson, C. (2002) "It doesn't Cost Anything to Ask, does It? The Ethics of Questionnaire-Based Research," *Journal of Medical Ethics*, 28(1): 41–44.

Fisher, C.B. (2003) *Decoding the Ethics Code: A Practical Guide for Psychologists*, Thousand Oaks, CA: Sage Publications.

Fisher, C.B. and Wallace, S.A. (2000) "Through the Community Looking Glass: Reevaluating the Ethical and Policy Implications of Research on Adolescent Risk and Psychopathology," *Ethics and Behavior*, 10(2): 99–118.

Food and Drug Administration (FDA) (1999) *Choice of Control Group in Clinical Trials* (Draft Guidance No. Docket No. 99D-3082), Rockville, MD: Food and Drug Administration.

Freedman, B. (1990) "Placebo-Controlled Trials and the Logic of Clinical Purpose," *IRB: A Review of Human Subjects Research*, 12(6): 1–6.

——(1987) "Scientific Value and Validity as Ethical Requirements for Research: A Proposed Explication," *IRB: A Review of Human Subjects Research*, 9(6): 7–10.

Gallant, D.R. (2002) "Qualitative Social Science Research," in R.J. Amdur and E.A. Bankert (eds) *Institutional Review Board: Management and Function* (pp. 403–06). Sudbury, MA: Jones and Bartlett.

Getz, K. and Borfitz, D. (2002) *Informed Consent: A Guide to the Risks and Benefits of Volunteering for Clinical Trials*, Boston, MA: CenterWatch.

Grisso, T. (1992) "Minors' Assent to Behavioral Research Without Parental Consent," in B. Stanley and J.E. Sieber (eds) *Social Research on Children and Adolescents: Ethical Issues* (pp. 109–27). Newbury Park, CA: Sage Publications.

Hadjistavropoulos, T. and Smythe, W.E. (2001) "Elements of Risk in Qualitative Research," *Ethics and Behavior*, 11(2): 163–74.

Haggerty, L.A. and Hawkins, J. (2000) "Informed Consent and the Limits of Confidentiality," *Western Journal of Nursing Research*, 22(4): 508–14.

Health Privacy Working Group. (1999) *Best Principles for Health Privacy: A Report of the Health Privacy Working Group*, Washington, DC: Health Privacy Project. Online available: www.healthprivacy.org/usr_doc/33807.pdf (accessed June 1, 2004).

Hoagwood, K. (1994) "The Certificate of Confidentiality at the National Institute of Mental Health: Discretionary Considerations in Its Applicability to Research on Child and Adolescent Mental Disorders," *Ethics & Behavior*, 4(2): 123–31.

Hoagwood, K., Jensen, P.S., and Fisher, C.B. (1996) *Ethical Issues in Mental Health Research with Children and Adolescents*, Mahwah, NJ: Lawrence Erlbaum Associates.

Humphreys, L. (1970) *Tearoom Trade: Impersonal Sex in Public Places*, Chicago, IL: Aldine.

Jenkins-Hall, K. and Osborn, C.A. (1994) "The Conduct of Socially Sensitive Research: Sex Offenders as Participants," *Criminal Justice and Behavior*, 21(3): 325–40.

Kelman, H.C. (1982) "Ethical Issues in Different Social Science Methods," in T.L. Beauchamp, R.R. Faden, R.J. Wallace, and L. Walters (eds) *Ethical Issues in Social Science Research* (pp. 40–98). Baltimore, MD: Johns Hopkins University Press.

Kelsey, J.L. (1981) "Privacy and Confidentiality in Epidemiological Research Involving Patients," *IRB: A Review of Human Subjects Research*, 3(2): 1–4.

Koocher, G.P. (2002) "Using the CABLES Model to Assess and Minimize Risk in Research: Control Group Hazards," *Ethics & Behavior*, 12: 75–86.

Koocher, G.P. and Keith-Spiegel, P.C. (1998) *Ethics in Psychology: Professional Standards and Cases*, 2nd edn, vol. 3, New York: Oxford University Press.

——(1990) *Children, Ethics, and the Law: Professional Issues and Cases*, Lincoln: University of Nebraska Press.

Korn, J.H. (1997) *Illusions of Reality: A History of Deception in Social Psychology*, Albany: State University of New York Press.

Lane, L.W., Cassel, C.K., and Bennett, W. (1990) "Ethical Aspects of Research Involving Elderly Subjects: Are We Doing More than We Say?," *The Journal of Clinical Ethics*, 1(4): 278–85.

Laufer, R.S. and Wolfe, M. (1977) "Privacy as a Concept and a Social Issue: A Multidimensional Developmental Theory," *Journal of Social Issues*, 33(3): 22–42.

Levine, R.J. (1988) *Ethics and Regulation of Clinical Research*, 2nd edn, New Haven, CT: Yale University Press.

Lustig, B., Coverdale, J., Bayer, T., and Chiang, E. (1993) "Attitudes Toward the Use of Deception in Psychologically Induced Pain," *IRB: A Review of Human Subjects Research*, 15(6): 6–8.

Macklin, R. (1982) "The Problem of Adequate Disclosure in Social Science Research," in T.L. Beauchamp, R.R. Faden, R.J. Wallace, and L. Walters (eds) *Ethical Issues in Social Science Research* (pp. 193–214). Baltimore, MD: Johns Hopkins University Press.

Margolis, L.H. (2000) "Taking Names: The Ethics of Indirect Recruitment in Research on Sexual Networks," *Journal of Law, Medicine & Ethics*, 28(2): 159–64.

Marshall, P.A. (1992) "Research Ethics in Applied Anthropology," *IRB: A Review of Human Subjects Research*, 14(6): 1–5.

Mastroianni, A.C. and Kahn, J. (2001) "Swinging on the Pendulum: Shifting Views of Justice in Human Subjects Research," *Hastings Center Report*, 31(3): 21–28.

Milgram, S. (1974) *Obedience to Authority: An Experimental View*, New York: Harper and Row.

——(1964) "Issues in the Study of Obedience: A Reply to Baumrind," *American Psychologist*, 19: 848–52.

National Bioethics Advisory Commission (NBAC) (2001) *Ethical and Policy Issues in Research Involving Human Participants*, Bethesda, MD: National Bioethics Advisory Commission.

——(1999) *Research Involving Persons with Mental Disorders that May Affect Decisionmaking Capacity*, Bethesda, MD: National Bioethics Advisory Commission.

National Commission for the Protection of Human Subjects of Biomedical and Behavioral Research (1979) *The Belmont Report: Ethical Principles and Guidelines for the Protection of Human Subjects of Research*, Washington, DC: Department of Health, Education, and Welfare.

National Institutes of Health (NIH) (2004) *"Ceritificates of Confidentiality Kiosk,"* Online available: http://grants.nih.gov/grants/policy/coc/ (accessed June 11, 2004).

National Library of Medicine (NLM) (1996) *"Current Bibliographies in Medicine: Confidentiality of Electronic Health Data, No. 95–10."* Rockville, MD: National Library of Medicine. Online available: http://www.nlm.nih.gov/pubs/cbm/confiden.html (accessed June 2, 2004).

National Research Council (NRC) (1997) *For the Record: Protecting Electronic Health Information*, Washington, DC: National Academy Press.

National Science Foundation (NSF) (2002) *"Interpreting the Common Rule for the Protection of Human Subjects for Behavioral and Social Science Research,"* Online available: http://www.nsf.gov/bfa/dias/policy/hsfaqs.htm (accessed January 26, 2005).

Oakes, M.J. (2002) "Survey Research," in R.J. Amdur and E.A. Bankert (eds) *Institutional Review Board: Management and Function* (pp. 428–33). Boston, MA: Jones and Bartlett.

Oakley, A. (1998) "Experimentation and Social Interventions: A Forgotten But Important History," *British Medical Journal*, 317: 1239–42.

Parrot, E.S. (2002) "Ethnographic Research," in R.J. Amdur and E.A. Bankert (eds) *Institutional Review Board: Management and Function* (pp. 407–14). Sudbury, MA: Jones and Bartlett.

Pattullo, E.L. (1982) "Modesty is the Best Policy: The Federal Role in Social Research," in T.L. Beauchamp, R.R. Faden, R.J. Wallace, and L. Walters (eds) *Ethical Issues in Social Science Research* (pp. 373–90). Baltimore, MD: Johns Hopkins University Press.

Pittenger, D.J. (2002) "Deception in Research: Distinctions and Solutions from the Perspective of Utilitarianism," *Ethics & Behavior*, 12(2): 117–42.

Pritchard, I.A. (2001) "Searching for 'Research Involving Human Subjects'. What is Examined? What is Exempt? What is Exasperating?," *IRB: Ethics & Human Research*, 23: 5–12.

Rada, R. (2003) *HIPAA@IT Essentials: Health Information Transactions, Privacy and Security*, 2nd edn, Baltimore, MD: HIPAA–IT.

Russell, C. (1999) "Interviewing Vulnerable Old People: Ethical and Methodological Implications of Imagining Our Subjects," *Journal of Aging Studies*, 13(4): 403–17.

Saint Louis University (2004) *"Disposal of Protected Health Information (PHI),"* Online available: http://www.slu.edu/hipaa/disposal_of_protected_health_information.pdf (accessed June 2, 2004).

Search Institute (2001) *Information Booklet. Search Institute Profiles of Student Life: Attitudes and Behaviors*. Minneapolis, MN: Search Institute. Online available: http://www.search-institute.org/surveys/AB_Info_Booklet.pdf (accessed May 27, 2004).

Shaw, I.F. (2003) "Ethics in Qualitative Research and Evaluation," *Journal of Social Work*, 3(1): 9–29.

Sieber, J.E. (2001a) "Privacy and Confidentiality as Related to Human Research in Social and Behavioral Science," in National Bioethics Advisory Council (ed.) *Ethical and Policy Issues in Research Involving Human Participants: Commissioned Papers and Staff Analysis*, vol. 2 (pp. N1–N50). Bethesda, MD: National Bioethics Advisory Committee. Online available: http://www.georgetown.edu/research/nrcbl/nbac/human/overvol2.pdf (accessed January 26, 2005).

Sieber, J.E. (2001b) *"Summary of Human Subjects Protection Issues Related to Large Sample Surveys"* (No. NCJ 187692), US Department of Justice.

——(1992) *Planning Ethically Responsible Research: A Guide for Students and Internal Review Boards*, vol. 31, Newbury Park, CA: Sage Publications.

——(1982a) "Deception in Social Research III: The Nature and Limits of Debriefing." *IRB: A Review of Human Subjects Research*, 5(3): 1–4.

——(1982b) "Kinds of Deception and the Wrongs They May Involve," *IRB: A Review of Human Subjects Research*, 4(9): 1–5.

Sieber, J.E. and Sorensen, J.L. (1992) "Conducting Social and Behavioral AIDS Research in Drug Treatment Clinics," *IRB: A Review of Human Subjects Research*, 14(5): 1–5.

Sieber, J.E. and Stanley, B. (1988) "Ethical and Professional Dimensions of Socially Sensitive Research," *American Psychologist*, 43(1): 49–55.

Sieber, J.E., Iannuzzo, R., and Rodriguez, B. (1995) "Deception Methods in Psychology: Have They Changed in 23 Years?," *Ethics & Behavior*, 5(1): 67–85.

Simon, G.E., Unutzer, J., Young, B.E., and Pincus, H.A. (2000) "Large Medical Databases, Population-Based Research, and Patient Confidentiality," *American Journal of Psychiatry*, 157(11): 1731–37.

Smith, M.W. (1995) "Ethics in Focus Groups: A Few Concerns," *Qualitative Health Research*, 5(4): 478–86.

Smythe, W.E. and Murray, M.J. (2000) "Owning the Story: Ethical Considerations in Narrative Research," *Ethics & Behavior*, 10(4): 311–36.

Soble, A. (1978) "Deception in Social Science Research: Is Informed Consent Possible?," *The Hastings Center Report*, 8(5): 40–46.

Speer, M.A. (2002) "Epidemiology/Public Health Research," in R.J. Amdur and E.A. Bankert (eds) *Institutional Review Board: Management and Function* (pp. 428–33). Sudbury, MA: Jones and Bartlett.

Stanley, B.H. and Guido, J.R. (1996) "Informed Consent: Psychological and Empirical Issues," in B.H. Stanley, J. Sieber, and G.B. Melton (eds) *Research Ethics: A Psychological Approach* (pp. 105–28). Lincoln, NE: University of Nebraska Press.

Stanley, B.H., Sieber, J., and Melton, G.B. (1996) *Research Ethics: A Psychological Approach*. Lincoln, NE: University of Nebraska Press.

Steinberg, J. (1983) "Social Research Use of Archival Data: Procedural Solutions to Privacy Problems," in R.F. Boruch and J.S. Cecil (eds) *Solutions to Ethical and Legal Problems in Social Research* (pp. 249–61). New York, NY: Academic Press.

Tangney, J. (2000) "Training," in B.D. Sales and S. Folkman (eds) *Ethics in Research with Human Participants*, Washington, DC: American Psychological Association.

Wallace, R.J., Jr (1982) "Privacy and the Use of Data in Epidemiology," in T.L. Beauchamp, R.R. Faden, R.J. Wallace, and L. Walters (eds) *Ethical Issues in Social Science Research* (pp. 274–91). Baltimore, MD: Johns Hopkins University Press.

Warwick, D.P. (1982) "Types of Harm in Social Research," in T.L. Beauchamp, R.R. Faden, R.J. Wallace Jr, and L. Walters (eds) *Ethical Issues in Social Science Research* (pp. 101–24). Baltimore, MD: Johns Hopkins University Press.

Weijer, C. (1999) "Protecting Communities in Research: Philosophical and Pragmatic Challenges," *Cambridge Quarterly of Healthcare Ethics*, 8: 501–13.

Wolf, L.E., Zandecki, J., and Lo, B. (2004) "The Certificate of Confidentiality Application," *IRB: Ethics & Human Research*, 26(1): 14–18.

7 When should research with infants, children, or adolescents be permitted?

Loretta M. Kopelman

Parents who learn that their child has schizophrenia may be expected to seek the best available care for this serious and chronic illness. Yet, these children are routinely undertreated because many interventions used for adults have not been tested on children (Findling *et al.* 1996; Quintana and Keshavan 1995). There are few well-tested options because, until recently, the prevailing view was that studies should be done first on competent adults and only later on vulnerable groups, such as infants, children, and adolescents (Dresser 1992). They were excluded from many studies in order to protect them, but the consequences were that they could not obtain investigational new drugs (INDs) or gain access to important studies. Thus, in attempting to protect them, these policies were sometimes causing them harm by denying them opportunities available to others and treating them unfairly.

Only a small number of treatments have been tested on children (AAP 1995; IOM 2004). For example, a majority of marketed drugs is unlabeled for pediatric populations. In addition, between 10 and 20 percent of research excludes pediatric populations without good reason (AAP 1995). If studies are not done with infants, children, or adolescents, however, it is hard to generalize results to them because they often react differently to drugs than adults. For example, a common antibiotic, chloramphenicol, caused death among neonates who could not tolerate this drug because their livers were so immature (NIH 1998). Studies done with adult participants have uncertain benefits for younger people. The very few pediatric studies that have been done have led some pediatricians to deny that evidence-based medicine exists in pediatrics.

During the HIV/AIDS epidemic, the practice of routinely excluding vulnerable groups from investigations came under scrutiny and was changed; it became clear that regulations were sometimes literally "protecting them to death" ("Expanded Availability..." 1990; Kopelman 1994; Merigan 1990). Participation in research can give individuals opportunities to gain access to programs or treatments that are otherwise unavailable to them. Research also benefits infants, children, or adolescents as a group. Medical science cannot assess their unique needs and reactions to interventions without systematic testing (Kopelman 2000, 2004a).

Legislators and the research community began addressing this problem, working to include all groups unless good scientific or ethical reasons can be made not to do so. Testing on pediatric populations should be done unless a case can be made that it would be unsafe, impractical, or otherwise unreasonable. For example, investigators might show that minors should be excluded because the area of study is irrelevant to their health or well-being or the information is already available, or they might show it is illegal to include them, or that the condition would be so rare in pediatric populations that it would be inappropriate to include them.

The enormous social utility of conducting research with children, however, should not mask the fact that some children have been harmed by participation in research. In one famous case, young retarded children at the Willowbrook State School on Staten Island in New York City were given hepatitis in order to study the disease (Kopelman 2000, 2004a). Investigators reasoned that the disease was endemic to this institution and so the children would get it in any case. But the children were exposed to considerable risk, often getting a more serious case of hepatitis than they might otherwise have gotten. Moreover, they got less protection than staff, who were routinely protected with gamma globulin. The children were put at risk in order to gain information that would benefit the general population. This study received harsh and lasting criticism (*Grimes v. Kennedy Krieger Institute* 2001a).

Thus, the dilemma at the heart of all pediatric research policy is How should society promote the best interest of children as a group through research while protecting the rights and welfare of the individual research subjects (Kopelman 2000, 2002, 2004a)? The same problem arises for adults, but they can help solve this dilemma for themselves by participating in research as informed and competent volunteers. They may even decide they want to take some risk in order to help develop generalized information that will benefit everyone. And as children get older, they may have increasingly greater capacity to learn about the study and decide for themselves whether they want to participate. For the most part, however, others must decide whether children will participate in research.

Clearly, a primary value must be to protect the infants, children, and adolescents who may participate in research (IOM 2004). At the same time, however, without research about the safety and efficacy of interventions, clinicians face another dilemma. If clinicians only use tested interventions, they severely limit treatment options for children. On the other hand, if clinicians use therapies that have not been well tested, their patients may be harmed by unanticipated results. Without studies, clinicians do not know if a promising intervention will be safe or effective or whether the testing may harm subjects.

As potential risks increase, it becomes harder to justify enrolling children in studies unless there is a direct benefit to them. This conclusion that greater risks require greater justification may be found in US pediatric research requirements and in many other guidelines (Kopelman 2000, 2004a; Kopelman and Murphy 2004). These rules will be reviewed after considering the moral basis for research with infants, children, and adolescents.

Moral principles underlying research policy

Moral principles offer general guidance about how to make practical choices, and several have become important for discussions in pediatric research policy. Rational consensus about the importance, meaning, and use of moral principles, within and between cultures, establishes points of agreement about our goals and thus offers opportunities to discuss and decide what course of action to take. Moral principles may be grounded in many ways depending upon one's moral stance (reason, experience, social interactions, prudence, religion, etc.) and it is not necessary to take a stance on this to use them. Following a series of controversies about research studies, policy makers, moral theorists, legal experts, and investigators sought a secure moral foundation for research policy; they developed the widely adopted and often-cited *The Belmont Report* (National Commission 1979) as a framework for research policy.

The drafters of *The Belmont Report* (National Commission 1979) organized moral considerations for research policy around three headings they also call "principles": *respect for persons* (analyzed to include the moral principles of autonomy and protection of vulnerable subjects), *beneficence* (analyzed to include the moral principles of beneficence, nonmalificence, and social utility), and *justice* (understood as distributive justice).

Respect for persons

The first principle, respect for persons, requires honoring persons' liberty and autonomy to make decisions and plan their own lives. An autonomous person is an individual capable of deliberation about personal goals and acting under the direction of such deliberation. While older adolescents may be as autonomous as most adults, clearly young children lack the capacity for autonomy. Thus, the drafters of *The Belmont Report* included under respect for persons the notion that vulnerable subjects, such as young children, have the right to added protections.

The requirement to respect persons serves as the basis for the duty to get consent from adults for participation in studies and permission from guardians to enroll children. It also is a basis for getting assent from children to the degree that is possible and desirable (some children do not want to assent), usually from children over 7. Investigators have a duty to gain informed consent from participants and permission from guardians. This involves making sure that their consent is (a) voluntary and not coerced or manipulated, (b) competent, and (c) informed. The general rule is that investigators need to provide information that a reasonable person would want in order to make a decision about whether or not to participate. The US Federal Regulations require that, at a minimum, subjects be told the study's nature, purpose, duration, procedure, foreseeable risks, and expected benefits. They must also be told about alternative procedures, how confidentiality is protected, and policy regarding compensation. In addition, participants or their guardians must be told whom to contact for questions or possible injuries. They must also be told of the voluntary nature of participation and of the right to withdraw from the study. Institutional Review Boards (IRBs) may require investigators to add additional information.

Children cannot generally protect their own well-being, so if children are to be enrolled in research, others must give permission. Parents' or guardians' permission is generally required for their children's participation in research. This is because, first, parents generally have the greatest knowledge about and interest in their own minor children. In addition, they have legal authority to make these and many other decisions for their minor children because they must deal with the consequences of the choices made (Buchanan and Brock 1989). Permission from parents in most cases is necessary for research. IRBs sometimes make exceptions allowing older adolescents to give informed consent for themselves if the study does not involve more than a minimal risk and could not be done otherwise.

Parental consent, however, is not sufficient since some parents/guardians might make imprudent decisions about enrolling their children in studies. Their intentions may be to foster their child's well-being and prevent, remove, or minimize harms, yet the complexity of research programs may mislead them. Enrolling children in research programs also requires layers of approval from others. Before children are allowed to participate, investigators, members of IRBs or ethics committees must also give approval. Their combined approval should help ensure that children are not abused, neglected, or exploited; however, additional regulatory protections are needed to protect the rights and well-being of children. These additional regulations are needed because while competent adults have the right to volunteer themselves for high-risk studies in order to gain knowledge, volunteering to put others in harm's way is not a right. Volunteering children for such studies could violate the parent's role in protecting the well-being of their children. Thus, parents cannot be permitted to enroll their children in high-risk studies just as they would themselves.

Even where parents, investigators, and institutional representatives agree that the child should be enrolled, they may have the responsibility to get the assent or agree-ment of the child to participate, especially if the study is not for the direct benefit of the child or there is some risk. Children as young as 7 years old are routinely consulted and their refusals should be definitive unless there is direct benefit to them for being in the study (IOM 2004). Securing the agreement of the child and the consent of the parent, then, is still not sufficient to justify enrollment of children in research, and an elaborate set of federal regulations must be followed in almost all research involving children.

Beneficence

The second principle identified by *The Belmont Report* is the principle of beneficence. This means that investigators will not intentionally harm subjects and that they will maximize possible benefits and minimize possible harms to participants. Under this principle, the drafters also acknowledged the social utility of research in advancing knowledge for diagnosis, treatments, advocacy, and prevention of disease. As ana-lyzed by the drafters of *The Belmont Report*, this statement of the principle of beneficence that combines nonmaleficence and social utility has an obvious tension. What benefits the group in doing a risky study may harm the subjects selected. For example, the Willowbrook hepatitis studies put young retarded children at risk by giving them a very serious disease, but a great deal of important information resulted from the study.

Infants, children, and adolescents are vulnerable and so need additional protection beyond what is provided to competent adults. Yet, protections for minors should not be so inflexible or set so high that research for them is unreasonably thwarted, or that they are kept from access to promising investigational drugs. If we say the child's well-being must always take precedence such that if there is any risk, studies must be prohibited, then many important and relatively safe studies will be halted on the grounds that one cannot be certain there is no risk whatsoever. For example, in order to obtain information on normal growth and development, information must be collected from children's records that do not, strictly speaking, present any risk of harm to the children. Nonetheless, we cannot call even this study absolutely risk-free since we might imagine that a loss of privacy might occur causing great damage to the child through discrimination or loss of self-esteem. The difficulty for research policy is, as noted, how to rank the study's risks of harm to participants, especially to children who cannot give consent for themselves, and the social benefits of doing the research. This question becomes especially acute when there is no direct benefit to the children. All research policy should address this issue.

Justice

The third principle identified by the drafters of *The Belmont Report* is that of justice.[1] This principle requires that participants be selected so that the burdens and benefits are distributed fairly. Certain groups should not be unfairly burdened either by being exposed to more risks of harm than others are or by being denied opportunities available to others. In the next section, I discuss a controversial study that raised issues about whether subjects had been unfairly singled out and coerced into participating in a study.

The SATURN study

The Student Athlete Testing Using Random Notification (SATURN) study was designed to study the effects of mandatory, random drug testing among high school students (Borror 2003; Chiodo *et al.* 2004; Goldberg *et al.* 2003). The goal was to compare high schools that had mandatory testing to those without such testing. In two separate Supreme Court decisions, the justices ruled that high schools could require student-athletes and others to undergo randomized drug testing as a precondition of participating in athletics or extramural activities (*Board of Education* 2002; *Veronica* 1995). The SATURN study sought to compare the schools electing to have mandatory drug testing programs with those that did not in order to see if the mandatory programs were effective. These programs are expensive and high school budgets are limited. Sometimes, their funding leads to the cutting of such important activities as art or music, so there should be evidence that they work.

There were two sorts of schools in the SATURN study. The *experimental schools* required that all student-athletes, at the beginning and end of the school year agree to mandatory, random drug testing and also complete name-linked but confidential questionnaires. A precondition for students to be in the sports program was for them to complete these questionnaires and submit to random testing for drugs and alcohol by urine samples collected by same-sex observers. The only option to avoid such questionnaires or testing was to withdraw from their sports program. If the student athletes tested positive, the parents and the schools would be notified, mandatory counseling would begin, and the students would not be able to participate in some or all of their sports events.

In contrast, the *control schools* did not have mandatory random drug testing and required that at the beginning and end of the school year, all students complete anonymous questionnaires that were not linked in any way to the students. The student-athletes were not singled out in any way.

Controversy swirled around this research study (Kopelman 2004b; Shamoo and Moreno 2004). Students and parents said that they were being pressured into participating in a research study as a precondition of being in the sports program. If correct, this would violate requirements that a research study must obtain the free, competent, and informed permission of parents and the assent of minors. They also objected that this research program caused confidentiality or privacy violations since the results were reported to the schools and the participants' parents, whether or not the students wanted either the schools or their parents to be told. Finally, they complained that the study was unfair because it was burdensome to one particular group of students in the effort to get information that would help everyone. That is, they said that the burdens upon the student-athletes were far greater than upon others. The choice of participating or leaving the school's athletic program was a heavy burden for students who sometimes viewed achievements in high school sports to be a ticket to college scholarships or career opportunities. Being denied these chances or being forced to participate in a research program to which they objected seemed coercive and unfair to them. In their review, Shamoo and Moreno (2004) concluded that SATURN violated well-established research policy including regulations about informed consent, confidentiality and privacy, and the just selection of research subjects.

The investigators conducting the SATURN study denied these accusations saying that they were simply monitoring the efficacy of different high school programs. They insisted that they were merely observing the efficacy of existing programs, not running them (Chiodo *et al.* 2004; Goldberg *et al.* 2003). The investigators and sponsors claimed that it was the schools, not the investigators themselves, who required student-athletes to participate in mandatory screening programs, had same-sex observers gather urine samples, and reported positive results to the schools or parents. These practices were school policy, the investigators argued, and SATURN was merely an independent research study observing and evaluating existing schools' programs.

Eventually the Department of Health and Human Services (DHHS) became involved and its Office of Human Research Protection (OHRP) stopped the study (Borror 2002). In their view, the investigators were not simply observers of different high school programs because the study's protocol was driving the high school testing and screening programs at the experimental schools. They reached this conclusion because of the random design of the programs, the nature of the drug testing, and the manner, collection, and evaluation of drug samples. In essence, OHRP agreed with the parents and the student-athletes, concluding that their "permission" and "assent" had been coerced, that their confidentiality and privacy had been compromised, and that unjust burdens had been placed on the student-athletes. The investigators and sponsors disagreed and tried to respond to these charges. Yet, in April 2003, OHRP concluded the investigators had not offered satisfactory answers to the charges (Borror 2003).

The SATURN study offers an example of how we may disagree about using moral principles and research regulations and also how we reach consensus. As more information became available, many reached the conclusion that the investigators, perhaps unintentionally, violated important policies. In the view of OHRP and many others, the SATURN study coerced participation, violated confidentiality and privacy rules, and was unfair in its selection of subjects (Borror 2003; Kopelman 2004b; Schamoo and Moreno 2004).

The SATURN study was a high profile and controversial investigation. Because it was carefully discussed, the SATURN study can serve as a paradigm to help set policy about what studies should be approved. It is important to include the public in the debate over what studies ought to be done with infants, children, and adolescents and the meaning and use of the federal regulations. In rare cases, however, sincere people of goodwill may continue to disagree, generally because they disagree about the relative importance of the values at stake or because they have factual disputes.

Research regulations

Most research guidelines distinguish different categories of pediatric research based upon whether the studies are designed to benefit the participants (as in research about cancer treatments) and whether they have more than a minimal risk of harm (see CIOMS 2002; Kopelman 2002, 2004a; US 45 CFR 46 1983; WMA 2001). In general, these rules require distinguishing studies that hold out direct benefits to subjects from those that do not; in addition, they stipulate that the greater the potential risk to children, the more rigorous the safeguards and the documentation about the probability and magnitude of benefits, harms, parental consent, and the child's assent. Many federal agencies and institutions receiving federal funding in the United States follow an elaborate set of pediatric regulations (IOM 2004; US 45 CFR 46 1983, 1991, 2002). The Institute of Medicine (IOM) has called for these rules to be adopted for all pediatric research in the United States (IOM 2004). I will focus upon these regulations in what follows. These regulations distinguish four categories of research; all require parental permission and the child's assent. They are sometimes known by their risk category and sometimes by their nomenclature in the Code of Federal Regulations (CFR), so I will list both.

46.404: Studies with no more than a minimal risk of harm

Research with no greater than a minimal risk may be authorized with IRB approval, even if it does not hold out direct benefit to individual research subjects, as long as it makes adequate provisions for consent from at least one guardian and, when appropriate, the assent of the child subject. Since the risk is low, direct benefit to individual research subjects does not have to be shown. For example, gathering information about children's growth from their medical records may not benefit them directly, but may be of enormous benefit to children as a group. Watching children stack blocks or identify animals from sound may not benefit participants directly, but help establish benchmarks of normal development. Minimal risk is understood as every day risks such as those encountered in routine physical, dental, or psychological examinations (Kopelman 2000, 2004a).

46.405: Studies holding out the prospect of direct benefit

Children are a distinctive group, and to evaluate standard or new therapies for them, some members of the group have to be included in studies. This second category of research allows IRBs to approve studies that have greater than minimal risk if it holds out the promise of direct benefit or therapy for them, and risks are justified because the intervention is at least as favorable for each subject as alternatives that are available. This category of research also requires parental consent and the child's assent when appropriate. Children, of course, have many unique problems, and the results from studies with adults may be inapplicable to children. To test the safety and efficacy of drugs for premature infants, premature infants will need to be subjects. Children with asthma, respiratory distress, or infections will have to be subjects in studies that evaluate the safety and efficacy of standard, innovative, or investigational drugs for these children.

46.406: Studies with no more than a minor increase over minimal risk

This category of research allows local IRBs to approve studies that have a minor increase over minimal risk even if the study does not hold out the prospect of direct benefit to the research participants. This requires the children in the study to have the condition or disorder under investigation. Consent from both parents is required if practicable, and the child's assent is needed if appropriate. To justify the higher level of risk, the study has to be similar to the children's actual or expected medical, dental, psychological, or educational experiences, as well as being likely to result in important information about the child's disorder and condition. "Minor increase over minimal risk" is undefined and so the problem with the concept of minimal risk is compounded (Kopelman 2000, 2004a). Given the recent legal ruling, *Grimes v. Kennedy Krieger Institute* (2001b), I have argued, however, that it should mean a minimal risk for these children with a disorder or condition, but no more than a minor increase over minimal risk for otherwise healthy and normal children without the conditions or disorders (Kopelman 2002).

46.407: More than a minor increase over minimal risk

Local IRBs cannot approve pediatric studies having more than a minor increase over minimal risk, but they can seek approval from the Secretary of HHS. To gain approval, it must represent a reasonable opportunity to understand, prevent, or alleviate a serious problem affecting the health or welfare of children. The Secretary of HHS can approve a study with more than a minor increase over minimal risk, but must first consult with a panel of experts about the study's value and ethics, gain parental permission, typically from both parents, and obtain the child's assent. In the United States, this category has also been used to review studies that have become controversial. Due to a variety of causes, including more financial and regulatory incentives to do pediatric research, there have been more appeals in the last three years than in the previous twenty since the regulations have been in existence (Kopelman and Murphy 2004).

Conclusion

One of the most difficult moral and social issues concerns when and under what circumstances infants, children, or adolescents should be permitted to be enrolled in research, especially when there is no anticipated benefit to them. A narrow road runs between too many protections and too few protections for children. The two extremes are entirely unsatisfactory. One extreme permits enrollment of infants, children, and adolescents in studies on the same basis as permitted for competent adults, with guardians giving permission. This extreme offers too little protection for infants, children, or adolescents. The other extreme forbids all studies with infants, children, or adolescents because they cannot give legally competent informed consent. (See the Nuremberg Code (1949) for an example of such a policy.) Others, near this end of the extreme, forbid any studies with any risk of harm unless there is a direct therapeutic benefit to the participating children. (See the pre-2000 World Medical Association (WMA) Declaration of Helsinki for an example of such a code.) Despite their good intentions to protect children, they would severely limit or even disallow studies on children (Kopelman 2000, 2004a). Because adults have different reactions to interventions, studies done with adults may be inapplicable to children. Drugs for childhood schizophrenia, diabetes, depression, infections, and respiratory distress should be tested for safety and efficacy on the children who get these drugs. Excluding vulnerable groups to protect their rights and welfare may have the opposite results. If good information about childhood disorders cannot be obtained for the pediatric population because of severe limiting of research, then it certainly does not promote their welfare, individually or collectively. Research rules, then, should honor duties to protect children's rights and welfare while giving them access to important opportunities and advancing knowledge for them as a group.[2] Herein lies the tension.

Notes

1 *The Belmont Report* can be faulted for not ranking these values, since they may conflict in just the same way that the principles can come into conflict. For example, there is great social utility in doing a study, yet it might be very harmful to subjects. Nonetheless, *The Belmont Report* served as a foundation for many research rules, including the need to get consent from competent adults or permission from them to enroll children as participants in research.

2 Copyright retained by Loretta M. Kopelman, PhD.

Bibliography

American Academy of Pediatrics (AAP), Committee on Drugs (1995) "Guidelines for the Ethical Conduct of Studies to Evaluate Drugs and Pediatric Populations," *Pediatrics*, 95(2): 286–94.

Beecher, H.K. (1966) "Ethics and Clinical Research," *New England Journal of Medicine*, 274: 1354–60.

Board of Education of Independence School District 92 of Pottawatomie County v. Earls 536 US 822 (2002).

Borror, K.C. (2003) "Office of Research Protection Department of Health and Human Services," April 17. Online available: http://ohrp.osophs.dhhs.gov/detrm_letrs/YR03/apr03c.pdf (accessed September 22, 2003).

——(2002) "Office of Research Protection Department of Health and Human Services," October 24. Online available: http://ohrp.osophs.dhhs.gov/detrm_letrs/YR02/oct02d.pdf (accessed September 22, 2003).

Buchanan, A.E. and Brock, D.W. (1989) *Deciding for Others: The Ethics of Surrogate Decision Making*, Cambridge, MA: Cambridge University Press.

Chiodo, G.T., Goldberg, L.G., and Moe, E.L (2004) "Orbiting SATURN: Countering Politically Charged Misinformation with Facts," *The American Journal of Bioethics*, 4(1): 43–48.

Council for International Organizations of Medical Science (CIOMS) (2002) International Ethical Guidelines for Biomedical Research Involving Human Subjects. Geneva, Switzerland: CIOMS.

Dresser, Rebecca (1992) "Wanted: Single, White Male for Medical Research," *Hastings Center Report*, 22(1): 24–29.

"Expanded Availability of Investigational New Drugs Through a Parallel Track Mechanism for People with AIDS and HIV-Related Disease" (1990). *Federal Register* 55, No. 98 (May 21): 20856–60.

Findling, R.L., Groevich, S.J., Lopez, I., and Schulz, S.C. (1996) "Antipsychotic Medications in Children and Adolescents," *Journal of Clinical Psychiatry*, 57(Supp. 9): 9–23.

Goldberg, L., Elliot, D.L., MacKinnon, D.P., Moe, E., Kuehl, K.S., Nohre, L., and Lockwood, C.M. (2003) "Drug Testing Athletes to Prevent Substance Abuse: Background and Pilot Study Results of the SATURN (Student Athlete Testing Using Random Notification) Study," *Journal of Adolescent Health*, 32(1): 16–25. (Erratum appears in *Journal of Adolescent Health*, 32(4): 325, Institute of Medicine of the National Academies of Science. *Ethical Conduct of Clinical Research Involving Children*. National Academies of Science, Washington, DC, 2004.)

Grimes v. Kennedy Krieger Institute, Inc. (2001a). 782 A.2d 807 (Md. 2001).

——(2001b). No. 128 (Md. October 11, 2001) (order denying motion for reconsideration).

Institute of Medicine (IOM) (2004). *The Ethical Conduct of Research Involving Children*, Washington, DC: National Academies Press.

Kopelman, L.M. (2004a) "Research Policy/II: Risk and Vulnerable Groups," in S.G. Post (ed.) *Encyclopedia of Bioethics*, 3rd edn (pp. 2365–72). New York: Simon & Schuster MacMillan.

——(2004b) "Adolescents as Doubly Vulnerable Research Subjects," *American Journal of Bioethics*, 4(1): 50–52.

——(2002) "Pediatric Research Regulations under Legal Scrutiny: *Grimes* Narrows Their Interpretation," *Journal of Law Medicine and Ethics*, 30: 38–49.

——(2000) "Children as Research Subjects: A Dilemma," *Journal of Medicine and Philosophy*, 25(6): 745–64.

Kopelman, L.M. (1994) "How AIDS Activists Are Changing Research," in D.C. Thomasma and J.F. Monagle (eds) *Health Care Ethics: Critical Issues* (pp. 199–209). Gaithersburg, MD: Aspen.

Kopelman, L.M. and Murphy, T.F. (2004) "Ethical Concerns about Federal Approval of Risky Pediatric Studies," *Pediatrics*, 113(6): 1783–89.

Merigan, T.C. (1990) "You Can Teach an Old Dog New Tricks: How AIDS Trials Are Pioneering New Strategies," *New England Journal of Medicine*, 323(19): 1341–43.

National Commission for the Protection of Human Subjects (1979) *The Belmont Report*, Report to the Secretary of the Department of Health, Education, and Welfare. (Now the Department of Health and Human Values.) Washington, DC: Government Printing Office.

National Institutes of Health (NIH) (1998) *NIH Policy and Guidelines on the Inclusion of Children as Participants in Research Involving Human Subjects*. March 6.

Nuremberg Code. Germany (Territory under Allied Occupation, 1945–1955: US Zone) Military Tribunals (1949) "Permissible Medical Experiments." In *Trials of War Criminals before the Nuremberg Tribunals under Control Law No. 10*, vol. 2. Washington, DC: US Government Printing Office. Online available: http://ohrp.osophs.dhhs.gov/irb/irb_appendices.htm (accessed July 1, 2004).

Pizzo, P.A. (1990) "Pediatric AIDS: Problems within Problems," *Journal of Infectious Diseases*, 161(2): 316–25.

President's Commission for the Study of Ethical Problems and Biomedical and Behavioral Research (1983) *Implementing Human Research Regulations*, Washington, DC: Government Printing Office.

Quintana, H. and Keshavan, M. (1995) "Case Study: Risperidone in Children and Adolescents with Schizophrenia," *Journal of the American Academy of Child & Adolescent Psychiatry*, 34(10): 1292–96.

Shamoo, A.E. and Moreno, J.D. (2004) "Ethics of Research Involving Mandatory Drug Testing of High School Athletes in Oregon," *The American Journal of Bioethics* 4(1): 25–31.

United States Code of Federal Regulations (CFR) (1991/2002) Protection of Human Subjects, Title 45 CFR 46.

——(1983) Title 45 CFR 46—see US Department of Health and Human Services: March 8, 1983, "Additional Protection for Children Involved as Subjects in Research," 48 *Federal Register 9,814–9,820* (March 8, 1983).

——(1981) Public Welfare Final Regulations Amending Basic HHS Policy for the Protection of Subjects. Title 45 CFR 46. *Federal Register 46*, No. 16: pp. 8366–92.

Veronica School District 47J v. Acton 515 US 646 (1995) Online available: http://supct.law.cornell.edu/supct/html/94–590.ZO.html (accessed September 22, 2003).

World Medical Association (WMA) (1964) *Declaration of Helsinki: Recommendations Guiding Medical Doctors and Biomedical Research Involving Human Subjects*, Adopted by the 18th World Medical Assembly, Helsinki, Finland. (Amended in 1975, 1983, 1989, 1996, and 2001.)

8 Biomedical research in the developing world

Ethical issues and dilemmas

David B. Resnik

Introduction

From the 1960s to the early 1990s, philosophers, theologians, physicians, lawyers, social scientists, and other writers in the emerging field of bioethics explored the problems and issues related to modern medical technology (Jonsen 1998). The highly influential foundational work in bioethics, Beauchamp and Childress' *Principles of Biomedical Ethics* (1979) discussed issues related to the appropriate use of technology, such as withdrawing or withholding artificial life support, assisted reproduction, organ transplantation, and genetic testing. While these issues can also arise in the developing world, most people in developing nations worry more about having access to *any* medical technology than about making appropriate use of medical technology.

Bioethicists did not pay much attention to the problems unique to the developing world until the 1990s, when people in the developed world became more aware of the dreadful effects of the human immunodeficiency virus (HIV) on the developing world. As we enter the twenty-first century, 45 million people worldwide have HIV, 30 million of which live in developing nations. Ninety-five percent of the 26 million people who have died from acquired immunodeficiency syndrome (AIDS) are from the developing world. It would cost more than $20 billion to treat the 6 million people in the developing world who are in immediate need of HIV medications. The developing world simply does not have sufficient economic, social, and biomedical resources to deal with this immense crisis. Few people in the developing nations have access to any medications to treat HIV. Very few developing countries have enough health-care professionals to deal with the HIV/AIDS crisis. Many people in developing nations also do not accept scientific theories about the causes of AIDS or public health recommendations designed to prevent the transmission of HIV, such as methods for practicing "safe" sex.

In response to the HIV/AIDS crisis, health-care providers, governments, and nongovernmental organizations (NGOs) from around the globe made heroic efforts to treat patients in the developing world and to try to prevent the spread of the disease. Biomedical researchers and health-care research organizations, such as the National Institutes of Health (NIH), the World Health Organization (WHO), and the Centers for Diseases Control (CDC), also began to develop new medications, treatment regimens, and public health programs to treat or prevent HIV. To achieve these goals, they recruited patients from developing countries to participate in

HIV/AIDS research conducted by researchers from the developed world. Pharmaceutical companies also began to sponsor clinical trials in developing countries and to market drugs to the developing world.

However, researchers, governments, and NGOs soon discovered that biomedical research in the developing world created some unique and challenging ethical dilemmas and problems. In order to deal with these issues, the WHO, the CDC, and the United Nations AIDS (UNAIDS) agency, in cooperation with local governments, began to work together to design clinical trials for studying HIV/AIDS therapies in the developing world. Peter Lurie and Sidney Wolfe (1997), two members of the Public Citizen's Health Research Group, ignited an international controversy when they published an article in the *New England Journal of Medicine* claiming that fifteen clinical trials developed by the CDC, WHO, and UNAIDS, some of which were sponsored by the NIH, were unethical. Marcia Angell (1997), the editor of the *Journal*, accused researchers of accepting ethical double standards and compared the studies to the infamous Tuskegee Syphilis Study. NIH Director Harold Varmus and CDC Director David Satcher (1997) wrote an article refuting the charges, and the debate continued. This chapter surveys some of the issues raised by Lurie, Wolf, and Angell, as well as some other ethical problems and dilemmas that arise in conducting biomedical research in the developing world. Although this chapter focuses on the disputed HIV studies, most of the issues raised by critics of these studies pertain to future research in the developing world.

Placebo controls

The controversial studies were clinical trials on methods for preventing perinatal (mother–child or vertical) transmission of HIV. In 1994, researchers developed a method for preventing perinatal transmission of HIV known as the 076 protocol. This method requires women to be tested for HIV infection early in pregnancy. If a woman tests positive for HIV, she receives oral and intravenous doses of the anti-retroviral drug zidovudine and foregoes breastfeeding. If the woman continues breastfeeding, she must continue to receive zidovudine while she breastfeeds. Infants also are given zidovudine for six weeks after birth. The 076 protocol reduces the rate of perinatal transmission of HIV from 25 percent to 8 percent. By the time the controversial studies took place, the 076 protocol had become the standard of care for pregnant women in developed nations, such as the United States (Resnik 1998).

At the time that the studies were conducted, very few people in the developing world had access to the 076 protocol, due to the high cost of the medications used to prevent HIV transmission and the lack of an adequate health-care infrastructure. Each year, more than 500,000 infants in the developing world acquire HIV from their mothers (De Cock *et al.* 2000). The 076 protocol requires the administration of about $800 worth of zidovudine, which is several hundred times the per capita spending on health care in some developing nations. The 076 protocol also requires a substantial health-care infrastructure to prescribe and administer zidovudine to the woman and her child, to provide prenatal care, and to conduct HIV tests. HIV researchers, in cooperation with local authorities, the CDC, WHO, and UNAIDS, determined that it was very important to try to develop an inexpensive and simple method for preventing the perinatal transmission of HIV. They wanted to know if it would be possible to significantly reduce the rate of mother–child transmission of HIV by administering $80 worth of zidovudine at specific times during pregnancy, labor, and after birth. Although the 076 protocol was the standard of care in developed nations, the goal was to develop a treatment that would be accessible and affordable for people in developing nations (Varmus and Satcher 1997). The researchers also wanted to determine whether a lower dose of zidovudine would be effective because they were concerned that pregnant women in developing nations are likely to have health problems, such as malnutrition and anemia, which could make it difficult for them to tolerate the higher doses of zidovudine required by the 076 protocol.

The researchers decided to conduct clinical trials that used placebo control groups in order to prove that a lower dose of zidovudine is more effective than nothing at all in developing world populations. The main reason researchers decided to include a placebo group in these disputed studies is that they believed that a placebo control group was required in order to achieve scientific rigor (Varmus and Satcher 1997). One of the fundamental principles of human research is that experiments should use scientifically valid methods and procedures (Emanuel *et al.* 2000; Levine 1986). Poorly designed experiments are unethical because they unnecessarily expose human subjects to research risks and waste resources. Virtually all research ethics codes require that experiments be well designed. The so-called gold standard for biomedical research, the randomized controlled clinical trial (RCT), achieves scientific rigor by using methods that help eliminate bias, such as randomization and blinding, as well as methods that are designed to yield statistically significant results, such as control groups and statistical power analysis (Elwood 1988).

A control group in a clinical trial could be an active therapy or an inactive one (a placebo). According to placebo orthodoxy, which is endorsed by the Food and Drug Administration, placebo control trials are more rigorous than active control trials. The reason researchers believe that placebo control trials are more rigorous than active control trials is that it is relatively easy to prove (or disprove) efficacy, using a small sample size, if one is only attempting to prove that a treatment is more effective than a placebo. In theory, one can still prove efficacy using an active control group, but this requires a larger sample size to achieve statistical significance (Djulbegovic and Clarke 2001; Emanuel and Miller 2001). Thus, the real reason why researchers often prefer placebo control trials to active control trials is that placebo control trials can yield quick, conclusive, and efficient results, while active control trials may take more time, cost more money, and yield results that are inconclusive. If there are financial, logistical, cultural, regulatory, or other factors that make it difficult to achieve the sample size needed for an active control trial, then it makes sense to conduct a placebo control trial. Moreover, since a placebo control trial may use fewer participants than an active control trial, it may expose fewer patients to the potential harms of an experimental treatment (Emanuel and Miller 2001).

In the disputed HIV studies, the researchers did not know whether one-tenth of the zidovudine used in the 076 protocol was more effective than no treatment at all.

The researchers decided that the most quick, efficient, and conclusive way of determining whether there are statistically significant differences between receiving a 10 percent dose of zidovudine and no treatment at all, was to compare the 10 percent dose to a placebo. Although it would have been possible to prove that a 10 percent dose is more effective than no dose at all without a placebo control group, this method would have required a much larger sample size to achieve statistically significant results, which would have taken more time and cost more money (Resnik 1998).

Less than a year after the ethical controversy erupted, researchers succeeded in proving that a 10 percent dose of zidovudine given in the last four weeks of pregnancy can reduce the perinatal transmission rate of HIV by 50 percent (DeCock *et al.* 2000). However, these successful results did not satisfy the critics, who argued that using placebos in these clinical trials was unethical because the research subjects also are patients in need of medical therapy. Patients in the placebo group did not receive any proven, effective therapy, whereas patients in the experimental group received some therapy. Defenders of the trials argued that the placebo group was needed to satisfy the demands of scientific rigor.

Clinical researchers who plan to use placebo control groups are caught between the horns of a dilemma: as researchers, they have an obligation to include a placebo group in order to achieve scientific rigor; as physicians, they have an obligation to not withhold treatment from their patients. According to a widely held view, the concept of clinical equipoise allows researchers to go between the horns of this dilemma: it is ethical to use a placebo group in research only when the medical community does not know whether the experimental treatment is more effective than a placebo. If there is a proven therapy for a disease, then all subjects with the disease should receive that proven therapy. When there is a proven medical therapy for a disease, researchers can compare different treatments, for example, experimental treatment versus standard treatment, but they cannot compare the standard treatment to a placebo (Freedman 1987). (See Miller and Brody 2003 for a critique of this view.) Many writers regard studies that use a placebo control group when a proven therapy exists as unethical because they subordinate the welfare of human subjects to scientific or social goals.

When these controversial HIV studies were conducted, the Declaration of Helsinki, a widely recognized international research ethics code, stated that all patients participating in biomedical research, including those in the control group, should receive the "best-proven diagnostic and therapeutic method," unless there is no proven diagnostic or therapeutic method. The Declaration also stated that the interests of science or society should not take precedence over the welfare of research participants (WMA 1996). Lurie and Wolf (1997) noted that the controversial studies violated the Declaration. Supporters of the controversial HIV research, such as Levine (1999), argued that the Declaration should be revised because it was seriously out of touch with the realities of clinical research. Levine objected to the requirement that all subjects receive the best-proven method unless there is no proven method. Critics of the HIV research, on the other hand, did not want to see this requirement eliminated.

As a result of this ethical controversy, the World Medical Association (WMA) decided to revise the Helsinki Declaration. The most recent version states that:

> [t]he benefits, risks, burdens, and effectiveness of a new method should be tested against those of the best current prophylactic, diagnostic, and therapeutic methods. This does not exclude the use of a placebo, or no treatment, in studies where no proven prophylactic, diagnostic, or therapeutic method exists.
>
> (WMA 2000: 3045)

As one can see, this statement in the Declaration is very similar to the previous one and it reaffirms the idea that patients/subjects should not receive a placebo if a proven therapy exists.

Thus, critics of these studies maintained (and continue to maintain) that they were unethical because they withheld effective treatments from participants in the placebo groups (Lurie and Wolfe 1997). Angell (1997) accused the researchers of accepting a double standard: one standard for the developed world and one for the developing world. If the HIV studies would be unethical in the developed world, then they should also be unethical in the developing world. If it is wrong to withhold a proven treatment in the developed world, then it is also wrong to withhold a proven treatment in the developing world (Angell 2000).

Defenders of the controversial studies argued that the obligation to provide research subjects with a proven therapy does not apply if the subjects do not already have access to that therapy. In the disputed HIV studies, subjects in the placebo group did not have access to any treatment for HIV, due to the high cost of medications and a poor health-care infrastructure. As a result of their economic and social conditions, the standard of care for these patients was no care at all. Thus, they were not being denied a treatment that would have been available to them. Moreover, the studies did not harm participants or increase their risk of transmitting HIV (Grady 1998). The questions of what constitutes (or should constitute) the standard of care for biomedical research in developing countries remain controversial. Some authors maintain that the standard of care should be local (Perinatal HIV Intervention in Research Developing Countries Workshop Participants 1999; Resnik 1998), while others hold that the standard of care should be universal (Lurie and Wolf 1997). (See London 2000 for further discussion.)

In response to this controversy, the Council for the International Organization of Medical Societies (CIOMS) also recently revised its Ethical Guidelines. The CIOMS (2002) Guidelines give researchers considerably more latitude when it comes to using control groups in clinical research in the developing world. According to Guideline 11:

> As a general rule, research subjects in the control group of a trial of a diagnostic, therapeutic, or preventive intervention should receive an established effective intervention. In some circumstances it may be ethically acceptable to use an alternative comparator, such as placebo or "no treatment." A placebo may be used: when there is no established effective intervention; when withholding an established effective intervention would expose subjects to, at most, temporary discomfort or delay in relief of symptoms; when use of an established effective

intervention as comparator would not yield scientifically reliable results and use of placebo would not add any risk of serious or irreversible harm to the subjects.

One important difference between the CIOMS Guidelines and the Helsinki Declaration is that the Guidelines only require patients to receive an "established effective intervention" instead of the "best proven" intervention. The Guidelines also list three exceptions to the rule that all subjects receive an effective therapy. The third exception would appear to apply to the disputed HIV studies, since use of an active control probably would not have yielded "scientifically reliable" results and use of the placebo did not cause any additional harm to the subjects, since they were not receiving any therapy prior to participating in the studies.

Informed consent

Informed consent is a pillar of ethical research (Emanuel *et al.* 2000). The Helsinki Declaration (WMA 2000) and the CIOMS (2002) Guidelines both require that individual research subjects (or their legal representatives) make an informed decision to participate in research. To make an informed decision, a person must have the ability to make an intelligent choice; they must have sufficient information; they must understand the information; and they must be able to make a free choice. Critics of the HIV studies also argued that the researchers violated these requirements of informed consent.

Some critics argued that the research subjects did not freely decide to participate in the studies because the studies presented them with coercive offers. Since the subjects did not have any access to health care, they were desperate for anything that could provide them with some help and protect their children from HIV infection (Tafesse and Murphy 1998). Although the subjects were vulnerable as a result of the disease and socioeconomic circumstances, they probably were still able to make a free choice to participate in the study. An offer is coercive if it presents a person with a threat rather than a mere opportunity. If a person will be made worse-off as a result of refusing an offer, then the offer is coercive (Brody 2002). For example, if a doctor threatens to stop treating a patient unless he participates in a research study, it would be a coercive offer. Since the disputed studies did not make the subjects who did not participate any worse-off as a result of their refusal, they were not coercive.

Other critics argued that the participants did not have enough information or did not understand the information they received. Interviews with some of the subjects who participated in these trials revealed that they did not understand the purpose of the research or the procedures that it involved. Many also believed that they were getting some type of treatment and did not understand that they were participating in a biomedical research (Resnik 1998). In response to the charges, proponents of the research argued that they made a sincere effort to provide individual research subjects with adequate information and that they attempted to help subjects understand that information. The disputed studies also provided participants with interpreters as well as informed consent documents translated into their own language.

Even though the disputed studies may have met the formal requirements of informed consent, they highlighted some of the linguistic and cultural difficulties with obtaining informed consent in the developing world. While interpreters can help researchers span linguistic divides, overcoming cultural differences is often more difficult (Levine 1991). As noted earlier, many people in developing nations do not accept scientific concepts, theories, and ideas. Many accept religious or supernatural explanations of health and disease and use alternative forms of treatment, such as healing rituals or herbal medicine. It can be difficult for subjects to understand the concept of a scientific experiment, let alone the methods and procedures needed to conduct a clinical trial.

Another important cultural difference between developed and developing nations is that most people in the developed world have a strong belief in individual rights. The individual's right to accept or refuse medical treatment provides the foundation for the legal and ethical doctrine of informed consent (Berg *et al.* 2001). People in developing nations may not embrace the developed world's emphasis on individual rights (Levine 1991). Indeed, a great deal of anthropological research on medical decision-making in developing countries indicates that the individual patient is not the locus of decision-making. Frequently, leaders of the family, the tribe, the community, or some other unit of social organization will make medical decisions instead of the individual patient/subject (Macklin 1999; Weijer and Emanuel 2000). What should a researcher do when these different decision-making paradigms conflict? Suppose that the leader of a tribe wants all of the members of the tribe to participate in a genetic study, but one member refuses. Or suppose that the leader of a tribe does not want members of the tribe to participate in a genetic study, but some members want to participate in it. To address conflicts between individual consent and community consent, several writers have proposed some methods for protecting the community's interests in biomedical research while respecting the individual's right to decide whether to participate in research (Newman 1996; Sharp and Foster 2000; Weijer 1999). The new CIOMS guidelines (2002) make some specific recommendations of how researchers should deal with these issues. Guideline 4 holds:

> In some cultures an investigator may enter a community to conduct research or approach prospective subjects for their individual consent only after obtaining permission from a community leader, a council of elders, or another designated authority. Such customs must be respected. In no case, however, may the permission of a community leader or other authority substitute for individual informed consent. ... Sponsors and investigators should develop culturally appropriate ways to communicate information that is necessary for adherence to the standard required in the informed consent process. Also, they should describe and justify in the research protocol the procedure they plan to use in communicating information to subjects. For collaborative research in developing countries the research project should, if necessary, include the provision of resources to ensure that informed consent can indeed be obtained legitimately within different linguistic and cultural settings.

Exploitation

Some of the critics of the disputed HIV studies argued that the studies were unethical because they exploited developing populations (Angell 1997; Crouch and Arras 1998). They were concerned that the benefits from the studies would accrue primarily to populations in the developed world, since populations in the developing world would not have access to results of the studies. They also argued that these studies would set a dangerous precedent that would lead to use of the research subjects as low-wage laborers for biomedical research that would benefit the developed world. Proponents of the studies, on the other hand, argued that they were not exploitative (Resnik 1998). Both sides of the dispute agreed that it is important to guard against the temptation to take advantage of vulnerable populations in the developing world for the sake of medical research or profit.

Although most people agree that biomedical research should not exploit populations in the developing world, there is little agreement about the meaning of "exploitation" (Macklin 2001). Exploitation in biomedical research involves taking unfair advantage of human subjects. Exploitation always involves at least one of three elements: disrespect, harm, or injustice (Resnik 2003). Disrespect occurs when researchers violate their subjects' dignity, autonomy, or privacy; harm occurs when researchers make their subjects worse-off as a result of participating in research; and injustice occurs when researchers do not employ adequate protections for vulnerable subjects or allocate the benefits and burdens of research unfairly. Exploitation, like other moral concepts, has degrees of gradation, ranging from highly exploitative practices, such as slavery, to minimally exploitative ones, such as pornography. In order to decide whether an exploitative research study is unethical, one must balance the wrongfulness of exploitation against other moral considerations, such as respect for individual rights or utility. Some minimally exploitative research may be ethical because other ethical concerns outweigh the duty to avoid exploitation (Brody 2002; Resnik 2003).

Since most researchers and ethicists agree on the importance of respecting human subjects and protecting them from harm, most of the disputes regarding exploitation in research center on questions about justice and fairness in research. A study that benefits subjects and treats them with respect might still be exploitative if it does not distribute the benefits and burdens of research fairly. The principle of justice in biomedical research requires that the benefits and burdens of research be distributed fairly (CIOMS 2002; The National Commission 1979; WMA 2000). Even though many researchers and research oversight agencies accept this general principle, disputes often arise concerning its application to particular situations. For example, is it fair to collect human genetic samples in order to develop a commercial database without giving subjects any financial compensation in return? Is it fair to provide subjects with free medications while they are participating in a clinical trial but to stop providing those medications once the trial ends?

To prevent exploitation and ensure that benefits and burdens are shared fairly, CIOMS (2002) Guideline 10 requires that:

- Research conducted in developing nations must be responsive to the health needs and priorities of that nation;

- The results of research, such as new knowledge or products, must be reasonably available to the population or community in which it is conducted;
- The distribution of the benefits and burdens of research must be equitable.

Participants in the 2001 Conference on Ethical Aspects of Research in Developing Countries (2002) made the following recommendations regarding benefit sharing:

- The research should provide fair allocation of benefits to participants and to the population before and after research, such as improvements in individual and public health, the provision of health services, economic development; the reasonable availability of medication, and the sharing of financial rewards of research;
- The research should be a collaborative partnership between researchers, sponsors, populations, and communities at all stages of development;
- Benefits agreements should be publicly accessible;
- There should be a process for consulting the community periodically about the research.

While many people accept these basic principles for avoiding exploitation, hard questions related to the specific details of research studies remain unresolved. For example, what does it mean for the results of research to be "reasonably available?" The disputed HIV studies developed a method for significantly reducing the risk of the perinatal transmission of the HIV for about $80 worth of zidovudine. This is a great improvement over an $800 treatment, but it is still too expensive for most HIV infected women in developing nations (Bloom 1998). Does this mean that the treatment was not reasonably available? In order to be "reasonably available," must the treatment be available to all patients who need it or only a significant percentage of patients who need it? Would $8 worth of zidovudine be a reasonably available treatment? If the treatment was not reasonably available when the research was completed but the researchers believed that it would be reasonably available when they proposed the study, does this mean that the research study was unfair and exploitative?

Another issue related to exploitation concerns providing medications and treatments to patients/subjects once the study has been completed. According to the Declaration of Helsinki, "At the conclusion of the study, every patient entered into the study should be assured of access to the best proven prophylactic, diagnostic, and therapeutic methods identified by the study" (WMA 2000: 3045). Many organizations have interpreted this rule to mean that research sponsors are responsible for paying for medication and treatment for research participants for an indefinite period of time after the study ends. Thus, if a patient/subject participates in a HIV clinical trial for six months, the sponsor would have to provide him or her with HIV medications for the rest of his or her life. While the goals of this policy are laudable, it may be unrealistic, since research sponsors may not be able to afford to provide free medications and treatment to patients/subjects for an indefinite period of time. If they cannot afford to provide the medication and treatment needed to conduct the study, then they may refrain from conducting the study at all. This is precisely what has happened at the National Institute of Allergy and Infectious Diseases (NIAID) as a result of this policy: the NIH has decided not to pay for the anti-HIV drugs for clinical trials sponsored by the NIAID (Cohen 2003).

Would it be exploitative to enroll a patient in a study and then stop providing medication to the patient once the study ends? To answer this question, one would need to consider whether stopping medications would be harmful, disrespectful, or unjust to the subject. Even if it would be exploitative to stop providing free medications once the study is completed, would it be unethical? Obviously, bioethicists need to explore these and related issues concerning justice and fairness in biomedical research in more depth (Cooley 2001; Macklin 2001).

Ethical relativism versus imperialism

As noted earlier, some critics, such as Angell (1997), argued that the disputed HIV studies implied a double standard: one set of ethical standards for the developed world and another for the developing world. According to these critics, there should be only one set of ethical standards for all biomedical research. The question of whether there are or should be a single set of rules for biomedical research that apply across the globe raises the meta-ethical issue of moral relativism (Macklin 1999; Resnik 1998). The double standard critique assumes that there should be one set of standards and that any deviation from those rules is unethical. In response to this charge, one could simply bite the moral relativism bullet and argue that different standards should apply to different populations, nations, or cultures. Indeed, defenders of the studies from host countries argued that bioethicists and researchers from developing nations were imposing their moral standards on developing countries by insisting that the clinical trials meet the ethical standards of the developed world (Mbidde 1998). They accused the critics of ethical imperialism. Developing countries, according to this argument, should be able to conduct their own clinical trials according to their own ethical standards. For those who do no accept moral relativism, there may be a way to avoid the dilemma of relativism versus imperialism. One might argue that there are ethical principles that apply across the globe, but that one must take local socioeconomic circumstances into account when interpreting and applying these principles (Macklin 1999; Resnik 1998). As we noted earlier, there is a great deal of cultural variation in practices relating to informed consent. There is also a great deal of variation relating to privacy, the role of religion in health care, access to health care, and the standard of care. Research studies may take these circumstances into account when interpreting and applying common ethical principles. To defend this alternative to relativism and imperialism, one must describe the relationship between principles and cases in more detail and explain how principles can guide moral judgment about specific cases. (For further discussion, see Beauchamp and Childress 2001.)

Patenting and drug development

The high cost of medications is a recurrent theme in nearly all of the ethical issues in research in the developing world. Indeed, if HIV medications were as cheap as aspirin, many of these disputed clinical trials would not have been conducted, and, if they were, they would probably not have included a placebo control because research sponsors would have been able to provide medications to the large number of participants needed to obtain scientifically rigorous data. The high cost of medications to treat infectious diseases, such as HIV, tuberculosis, and malaria, is a serious impediment to access to health care in the developing world (Resnik 2001). Another serious impediment is the fact that research sponsors are generally not interested in funding studies related to the health problems of the developing world. Many pharmaceutical companies would rather invest their resources in developing a new "blockbuster" drug to treat impotence, hypertension, or depression, than to invest in developing a vaccine for HIV or malaria. According to some estimates, 90 percent of the world's medical research dollars are spent to address 10 percent of the world's burden of disease (Benatar 2000).

Intellectual property laws and treaties have a direct bearing on the high cost of medications as well as the lack of research on the problems of the developing world. Pharmaceutical companies rely on intellectual property laws to protect their proprietary interests and obtain a reasonable return on research and development (R&D) costs. Most countries provide twenty years of patent protection for new and useful inventions. During the patent period, the patent holder has exclusive rights over the invention: no one can make, use, or commercialize the patented invention without permission of the patent holder. Once the patent expires, anyone can make, use, or commercialize the invention. It takes, on average, 10–12 years and $800 million to develop a new drug, test it, and bring it the market. Thus, pharmaceutical companies have about 8–10 years of patent protection during which they can recoup their R&D expenses. Once the patent expires, other companies can make generic versions of the drug. The company will be able to maintain its trademarked name for the drug, but other companies will be able to enter the market. As a result, competition will increase and the price will fall.

Sovereign nations have their own intellectual property laws. In order for an inventor to obtain patent protection in any particular nation, he must apply for a patent in that nation. When a pharmaceutical company decides to market a drug internationally, it will seek patent protection in different countries across the globe. Even though the intellectual property laws of different nations apply only within those nations, intellectual property treaties, such as the Trade Related Aspects of Intellectual Property Rights (TRIPS) agreement, provide for international harmonization of intellectual property protection. Members of the World Trade Organization (WTO), which includes many developing and developed nations, have signed the TRIPS agreement. TRIPS provides for:

- Minimal standards of protection for patents and copyrights;
- A forum for mediating disputes;
- Rules that require signatory countries to not undermine intellectual property protection of other signatory countries;

- Parallel importing from inventions from other signatory countries;
- A national emergency exception: a signatory country may override a patent (through a mechanism known as compulsory licensing) to deal with a national emergency.

(Nerozzi 2002)

In order to help promote access to HIV medications, many developing countries have considered taking steps to work with or around the TRIPS agreement, such as importing drugs from countries that do not honor the agreement or invoking the emergency exception. When South Africa adopted legislation to authorize the importing of cheap HIV medications and compulsory licensing, several pharmaceutical companies, including Merck, Glaxo-Wellcome, and Bristol Myers-Squibb, brought a lawsuit against South Africa. The companies later dropped the lawsuit in response to intense domestic and international pressure (Barnard 2002). As a result of the dispute, many pharmaceutical companies have agreed to lower the prices of HIV medications in developing nations and have instituted programs to provide free medications (Resnik 2001). This gesture by the pharmaceutical industry has helped to alleviate the problem of access to HIV medications, but it has not solved it.

Many doctors, researchers, and other critics are horrified that economic interests would take priority over the need to address a health-care crisis. According to these critics, all medications should be manufactured and sold as cheaply as possible so that as many people as possible can have access to them. Pharmaceutical companies and world governments have blood on their hands for conspiring to elevate the price of these vital medications (Justo 2002).

But the problem is not as simple as one might suppose. If pharmaceutical companies do not have adequate intellectual property protection in the developing world, they will not invest funds in developing new drugs for the developing world, and they will not establish markets in the developing world. Pharmaceutical and biotechnology companies currently fund more than 60 percent of the biomedical research conducted in the world. Private companies spent more than $40 billion on biomedical research and development in the United States in 2001 as compared to about $20 billion by the NIH (Resnik 2001). If pharmaceutical companies do not have patent protection for medications used to treat or prevent diseases of special concern to the developing world, they will invest their R&D funds in drugs for the developed world.

The dispute about patents on HIV medications raises important issues concerning access to health-care, justice, the economics of drug development, the social responsibilities of pharmaceutical companies, and international trade (Resnik 2001). The solution to this complex conflict requires cooperation and collaboration between pharmaceutical companies, researchers, the governments of developing and developed nations, and NGOs, to fund R&D on health problems that affect the developing world and to increase the affordability and accessibility of essential medications (Cohen and Illingworth 2003; Daniels 2001). Since poverty, famine, ignorance, war, and oppression are the root causes of many of the health problems that affect the developing world, to achieve long-term progress in reducing the impact of HIV on the developing world, developed nations should provide developing nations with the aid that they need to improve their health-care infrastructures, their economic, political, and legal systems, and their public understanding of biomedicine and the transmission and prevention of disease.

Bibliography

Angell, M. (2000) "Investigators' Responsibilities for Human Subjects in Developing Countries," *New England Journal of Medicine*, 342: 967–69.

——(1997) "The Ethics of Clinical Research in the Third World," *New England Journal of Medicine*, 337: 847–49.

Barnard, D. (2002) "In the High Court of South Africa, Case No. 4138/98: The Global Politics of Access to Low-Cost AIDS Drugs in Poor Countries," *Kennedy Institute of Ethics Journal*, 12: 159–74.

Beauchamp, T. and Childress, J. (2001) *Principles of Biomedical Ethics*, 5th edn, New York: Oxford University Press.

——(1979) *Principles of Biomedical Ethics*, New York: Oxford University Press.

Benatar, S. (2000) "Avoiding Exploitation in Clinical Research," *Cambridge Quarterly of Healthcare Ethics*, 9: 562–65.

Berg, J., Appelbaum, P., Lidz, C., and Parker, L. (2001) *Informed Consent: Legal Theory and Clinical Practice*, 2nd edn, New York: Oxford University Press.

Bloom, B. (1998) "The Highest Attainable Standard: Ethical Issues in AIDS Vaccines," *Science*, 279: 186–88.

Brody, B. (2002) "Philosophical Reflections on Clinical Trials in Developing Countries," in R. Rhodes, M. Battin, and A. Silvers (eds) *Medicine and Social Justice* (pp. 197–210). New York: Oxford University Press.

Cohen, J. (2003) "Drug Trials with the Drugs?," *Science*, 300: 1212–13.

Cohen, J. and Illingworth, P. (2003) "The Dilemma of Intellectual Property Rights for Pharmaceuticals: The Tension between Ensuring Access of the Poor to Medicines and Committing to International Agreements," *Developing World Bioethics*, 3: 27–48.

Cooley, D. (2001) "Distributive Justice and Clinical Trials in the Third World," *Theoretical Medicine and Bioethics*, 22: 151–67.

Council for International Organizations of Medical Sciences (CIOMS) (2002) "*International Ethical Guidelines for Biomedical Research Involving Human Subjects*," Online available: http://www.cioms.ch/frame_guidelines_nov_2002.htm (accessed November 15, 2004).

Crouch, R. and Arras, J. (1998) "AZT Trials and Tribulations," *Hastings Center Report*, 28(6): 26–34.

Daniels, N. (2001) "Social Responsibilities and Global Pharmaceutical Companies," *Developing World Bioethics*, 1: 38–41.

De Cock, K., Fowler, G., Mercier, E., de Vincenzi, I., Saba, J., Hoff, E., Alnwick, J., Rogers, M., and Shaffer, N. (2000) "Prevention of Mother-to-Child HIV Transmission in Resource-Poor Countries: Translating Research into Policy and Practice," *Journal of the American Medical Association*, 283: 1175–82.

Djulbegovic, B. and Clarke, M. (2001) "Scientific and Ethical Issues in Equivalence Trials," *Journal of the American Medical Association*, 285: 1206–08.

Elwood, M. (1988) *Causal Relationships in Medicine*, Oxford: Oxford University Press.

Emanuel, E. and Miller, F. (2001) "The Ethics of Placebo-Controlled Trials: A Middle Ground," *New England Journal of Medicine*, 345: 915–19.

Emanuel, E., Wendler, D., and Grady, C. (2000) "What Makes Clinical Research Ethical?," *Journal of the American Medical Association*, 283: 2701–11.

Freedman, B. (1987) "Equipoise and the Ethics of Clinical Research," *New England Journal of Medicine*, 317: 141–45.

Grady, C. (1998) "Science in the Service of Healing," *Hastings Center Report*, 28(6): 34–38.

Jonsen, A. (1998) *The Birth of Bioethics*, New York: Oxford University Press.

Justo, L. (2002) "A Patent to Kill? Comments on Resnik," *Developing World Bioethics*, 2: 82–86.

Levine, R. (1999) "The Need to Revise the Declaration of Helsinki," *New England Journal of Medicine*, 341: 531–34.

——(1991) "Informed Consent: Some Challenges to the Universal Validity of the Western Model," *Law, Medicine, and Healthcare*, 19: 207–13.

——(1986) *Ethics and Regulation of Clinical Research*, 2nd edn, New Haven, CT: Yale University Press.

London, A. (2000) "The Ambiguity and the Exigency: Clarifying 'Standard of Care' Arguments in International Research," *Journal of Medicine and Philosophy*, 25: 379–97.

Lurie, P. and Wolfe, S. (1997) "Unethical Trials of Interventions to Reduce Perinatal Transmission of the Human Immunodeficiency Virus in Developing Countries," *New England Journal of Medicine*, 337: 853–56.

Macklin, R. (2001) "After Helsinki: Unresolved Issues in International Research," *Kennedy Institute of Ethics Journal*, 11: 17–36.

——(1999) *Against Relativism: Cultural Diversity and the Search for Universals in Medicine*, New York: Oxford University Press.

Mbidde, E. (1998) "Bioethics and Local Circumstances," *Science*, 279: 155.

Miller, F. and Brody, H. (2003) "A Critique of Clinical Equipoise: Therapeutic Misconception and the Ethics of Clinical Trials," *Hastings Center Report*, 33(3): 19–28.

National Commission for the Protection of Human Subjects of Biomedical and Behavioral Research (1979) "The Belmont Report: Ethical Principles and Guidelines for the Protection of Human Subjects of Research," Online available: http://ohsr.od.nih.gov/guidelines/belmont.html (accessed November 17, 2004).

Nerozzi, M. (2002) "The Battle over Life-Saving Pharmaceuticals: Are Developing Countries Being 'TRIPped' by Developed Countries?," *Villanova Law Review*, 47: 605–41.

Newman, A. (1996) "Drugs Trials, Doctors, and Developing Countries: Toward a Legal Definition of Informed Consent," *Cambridge Quarterly of Healthcare Ethics*, 5: 387–99.

Participants in the 2001 Conference on Ethical Aspects of Research in Developing Countries (2002) "Ethics: Fair Benefits for Research in Developing Countries," *Science*, 298: 2133–34.

Perinatal HIV Intervention Research in Developing Countries Workshop Participants (1999) "Science, Ethics, and the Future of Research into Maternal Infant Transmission of HIV-1," *Lancet*, 353: 832–35.

Resnik, D. (2003) "Exploitation in Biomedical Research," *Theoretical Medicine and Bioethics*, 12: 197–224.

——(2001) "Developing Drugs for the Developing World: An Economic, Legal, Moral, and Political Dilemma," *Developing World Bioethics*, 1: 11–32.

——(1998) "The Ethics of HIV Research in Developing Nations," *Bioethics*, 12: 286–306.

Sharp, R. and Foster, W. (2000) "Involving Study Populations in the Review of Genetic Research," *Journal of Law, Medicine, and Ethics*, 28: 41–51.

Tafesse, E. and Murphy, T. (1998) "Ethics of Placebo-Controlled Trials of Zidovudine to Prevent the Perinatal Transmission of HIV in the Third World," *New England Journal of Medicine*, 338: 838.

Varmus, H. and Satcher, D. (1997) "Ethical Complexities of Conducting Research in Developing Countries," *New England Journal of Medicine*, 337: 1000–05.

Weijer, C. (1999) "Protecting Communities in Research: Philosophical and Pragmatic Challenges," *Cambridge Quarterly of Healthcare Ethics*, 8: 501–13.

Weijer, C. and Emanuel, E. (2000) "Protecting Communities in Biomedical Research," *Science*, 289: 1142–44.

World Medical Association (WMA) (2000) "Declaration of Helsinki: Ethical Principles for Medical Research Involving Human Subjects," *Journal of the American Medical Association*, 284: 3043–45.

——(1996) "Declaration of Helsinki," reprinted in J. Sugarman, A. Mastroianni, and J. Kahn (eds) *Ethics of Research with Human Subjects* (pp. 14–18). Frederick, MD: University Publishing Group.

9 Financial conflicts of interest and the human passion to innovate

Mark J. Cherry

Medical research and the human condition

In medicine one must abandon the presupposition that customary or accepted treatments are good simply because they are customary and accepted, and critically examine the standard of care together with new alternatives. Thorough and critical scientific research is integral to reigning in the untutored human desire to ameliorate pain and suffering so that medical treatments do more good than harm. It is often difficult to know truly in medicine, however. Problems such as spontaneous remissions and natural cures, physician remembrance of therapeutic triumphs more clearly than failures, the placebo effect, and the psychology of discovery, each distorts judgments of a treatment's efficacy. At times and in various ways, physicians, scientists, and patients see what they anticipate. The medical field compounds these challenges with the all too human impulse to help those in need. Yet, as the history of medicine pays witness, many interventions do more harm than benefit. Human suffering caused by ill-founded, but well-meaning, treatments has been significant. Scientific research, including clinical studies on human subjects, is central to the advancement of medical practice—including the development of advanced, more efficient and effective, pharmaceuticals and medical devices.

Since information gleaned through pharmaceutical research and clinical trials shapes diagnostic and therapeutic decisions, the concern is that for such information to be of significant value, it should not be subject to extraneous secondary considerations. Conflicts of interest in research arise when a researcher's judgment regarding a primary interest, such as scientific knowledge, is or may be unduly influenced by a secondary interest, such as financial gain, political viewpoints, or career advancement (Medical Research Council 2003: 208; see also Thompson 1993: 573).[1] Physicians who are both researchers and clinicians, for example, have competing commitments. The primary goal of clinicians is generally doing what is best for one's patients within certain side constraints, such as individual consent, institutional policy, and resource availability. Clinicians recommend treatments and interventions based on what they believe is in the best interests of their particular patients. The primary goal of researchers, in contrast, is the discovery of answers to research questions. Researchers are constrained in how they may utilize subjects who may or may not benefit from the study design; however, the objective in a scientific inquiry is to follow a protocol to obtain data, to test a hypothesis, and to contribute to the base of scientific knowledge.

The researcher's actions and decisions are not based on or directed primarily toward the interests of individual patient subjects.[2] When clinician-researchers enroll their own patients into clinical trials, especially if the studies include a placebo-controlled arm—in which subjects do not receive potentially beneficial medicine—a conflict of professional roles emerges since study subjects are not patients in a strict sense.[3] Other conflicts may emerge when researchers perceive certain conclusions as supporting particular moral judgments or sociopolitical points of view, or personal financial gain.[4]

Much of the literature has focused on identifying and managing financial conflicts of interest, in particular, to assess the extent of the scientific compromise. Many perceive financial gain as a secondary interest that overwhelms or distorts scientific professional judgment.[5] Critics argue that per capita payments and finder's fees, for example, may harm research subjects and negatively affect the patient/physician relationship;[6] that gifts from industry sponsors, such as discretionary funds, support for students, research equipment, stock ownership, trips to industry conferences, or honoraria for speaking engagements may bias interpretation and reporting of results.[7] Many charge that the financial interests of investigators:

1   dominate or appear to dominate the primary goal of obtaining objective research data for the future treatment of patients:
2   lower scientific standards;
3   impact research priorities, that is, change decisions about what to study:[8]
4   delay publication of important results, while researchers or others (e.g., pharmaceutical companies or universities) pursue patent and other legal protections:
5   unconsciously distort data or lead to outright fraud;
6   result in loss of public confidence in medicine and clinical research; and
7   negatively affect patient care.[9]

The forces of for-profit pharmaceutical development and clinical medical research, commentators urge, bring on more harm than benefit. The literature does not usually regard the profit motive as leading to the wise use of resources, the protection of human subjects, and the development of high quality and innovative pharmaceuticals and medical devices. Rather, commentators more typically view profiting from medical research, such as the development of pharmaceuticals and medical devices, as morally suspect.

As will be explored, financial conflicts of interest have drawn significant recent attention because of a changing research environment that encourages collaboration between commercial industry and the nonprofit academy. However, the ubiquitous calls for reform and regulation risk enacting facile and oversimplified solutions to what is a complex problem. As I will argue, to assess the risks involved in accepting financing from commercial interests, one must also consider the background risks involved in a medicine bereft of the significant bolus of funds the commercial industry provides to support both patient treatment and medical progress through the development of pharmaceuticals and medical devices. Insofar as commercial financing leads to greater innovation of lifesaving and life-enhancing pharmaceuticals and medical devices than alternative strategies, then constraining product development though the restriction of financial rewards and profits, or limitations on patent protections, may hinder the pace of innovation. This would in turn lead to significant harms to both present patients and future persons.

Some problematic cases

The practice of free and informed consent for health care in the United States is nested in a cultural affirmation of the moral importance of respecting the choices of individuals. It recognizes as well the difficulty of knowing what it means to choose correctly in a secular, morally pluralistic society. Absent an agreement regarding the requirements of God or the demands of moral rationality, individuals have been identified within rather broadside constraints as the source of authority over themselves and as the best judges of what choices are in their own interest (Cherry and Engelhardt 2004; Engelhardt 1996). The challenge is that certain economic arrangements appear to divorce the physician's financial interests from the patient's medical interests, influencing the treatments suggested and the information provided by physicians to patients, thereby affecting the adequacy of the patient's consent to treatment. As a result, many perceive the economics of medical research as presenting a pervasive challenge to the traditional fiduciary obligations of physicians (Khushf 1998).[10]

Consider the case of Thomas Parham, whose physician allegedly encouraged him to participate in a clinical trial studying a new drug designed to shrink enlarged prostates. While Mr Parham had not had any prostate difficulties, his physician allegedly stated that the drug might prevent future problems. A year earlier, Mr Parham had been hospitalized for a chronic slow heart rate, which should have disqualified him from participating in the study. However, his physician sought an exemption from the drug company. After Mr Parham began taking the study drugs, he evidently experienced fatigue, a symptom of a slow heart rate. Eventually, his physician hospitalized Mr Parham, and implanted a pacemaker to address the heart problem. What became clear only after the fact was that Mr Parham's physician was receiving $1,610 for each patient he enrolled in the study. While the pharmaceutical company designed this fee to cover study expenses, it was allegedly sufficient to provide the recruiting physician with a reasonable profit per enrolled patient (see Goldner 2000).

In a similar case, Jesse Gelsinger, an 18-year old, died following his participation in a gene study at the University of Pennsylvania's Institute for Human Gene Therapy. Gelsinger suffered from a rare liver disorder that he managed with a combination of special drugs and diet. Food and Drug Administration (FDA) investigators concluded that researchers placed him on the scientific protocol and gave him an infusion of genetic material even though his liver was not functioning adequately to meet the minimal level required under study criteria. The FDA further criticized the study for failure to notify the FDA of severe side effects experienced by prior subjects that may have been sufficient to halt the study, failure to notify the FDA of the deaths of four monkeys that were tested using similar treatments, failures in Gelsinger's consent form to notify him of such potential harms, as well as the inability to document that all research subjects had been informed of the risks and benefits of the protocol. The FDA documented other cases of patients who should have been considered ineligible because they were too ill to meet the protocol's standards. Eventually, the FDA suspended all gene therapy studies at this Institute. Among the FDA's criticisms, it emerged that the director of the Institute, James M. Wilson, owned stock in Genovo, the company financing the research. Moreover, Wilson and the former dean of the medical school owned patents on aspects of the procedure. Wilson admitted that he would gain $13.5 million in stock from a biotechnology company in exchange for his shares of Genovo and that the University had some $1.4 million in equity interest in Genovo. According to their agreement, Genovo would receive any rights to gene research discoveries at the Institute in exchange for financial support (see Goldner 2000).

The concern is that Parham and Gelsinger do not represent isolated cases; rather, these cases are examples of a more pervasive problem, especially as the research environment has changed in ways that blur the distinction between academic and commercial research, leading to significant financial conflicts of interest to the detriment of human subjects and scientific medicine.

Strategies for controlling conflicts of interest

Controlling conflicts of interest is an issue of institutional and professional virtue and character. The usual practice is to rely on the use of scientific criteria, including publication of data and methods of investigation, through the peer review process, to sustain the practice of impartial professional scientific investigation. Still, the federal government, most states, and academic institutions have developed conflict-of-interest policies to monitor university and researcher financial entanglements. Commentators typically place conflicts of financial interest within three categories: those that are small enough that they are unlikely to affect research, those that are manageable, and those that regulations should prohibit or that preclude the researcher from engaging in the research. While the design of clinical trials typically avoids fraud—for example, in that random assignment is made to various treatment arms; in that the trial is double blinded (i.e., that neither the researcher nor the patient know which treatment the patient is receiving); in that independent groups often gather and analyze data—there is still opportunity, as Baruch Brody points out, for the investigator's secondary interests to affect the study's design, conduct, and data analysis (1996: 407–17; see also Lo *et al.* 2000).[11]

The most popular strategy for reducing conflicts of interest has been the disclosure of financial holdings and arrangements that may present potential conflicts to the institutional review board (IRB) or an institutional conflicts of interest committee, department chair, university official, or legal counsel. At times, even public disclosure is specified, such as in public presentations or publication of research. Policies frequently prohibit research, if such economic entanglements exceed a certain threshold amount, usually $10,000. Disclosure requirements generally apply to equity holdings, stock and stock options, as well as income from salary, honoraria, and consulting fees. Such reporting usually applies to the researchers' assets as well as to the holdings of their spouses and dependent children, although some institutions request disclosure from parents, siblings, and adult children as well.[12] Other methods include oversight of the research, either by a supervisor or a committee, divestiture of financial entanglements, or modification of research. Universities have at times assigned a different faculty member to lead a research project or requested that the faculty member for whom there exists a potential conflict take a leave of absence (Cho *et al.* 2000).

The federal Office of Research Integrity of the US Department of Health and Human Services (DHHS) guidelines for managing conflicts of interest and promoting objectivity in research, for example, requires that all institutions wishing to do research with public health service funds maintain and enforce a written conflict of interest policy. Institutional responsibility includes collecting financial disclosure statements from each investigator of interests that would reasonably be assumed to constitute a conflict of interest, and to update such disclosures periodically during the period of the award. Such conflicts might include "anything of monetary value, including but not limited to, salary or other payments for services (e.g., consulting fees or honoraria); equity interests (e.g., stocks, stock options or other ownership interests); and intellectual property rights (e.g., patents, copyrights and royalties from such rights)" (ORI 2000). Researchers are not required to disclose equity, salary, and other financial arrangements that do not exceed $10,000.[13]

Similarly, the Association of American Universities' task force on conflicts of interest recommends that universities assess the adequacy of their procedures for managing conflicts of interest so that risks to the objectivity of research are minimized. They urge that universities, together with their research partners—commercial industry or governmental agencies—understand themselves as fully accountable for the design and integrity of their research. Institutionally, the disclosure process allows a university to assess and monitor such concerns. Many have developed review committees to assess potential conflicts, consider costs and benefits, and make recommendations regarding appropriate actions. The review committee judges, for example, whether to modify the financial arrangements, to establish a process to monitor the integrity of the research, to establish procedures to insulate financial decision-making from research decision-making, or to recommend that the research be prohibited (Hasselmo 2002: 426).

Insofar as the protocol involves research on human subjects, the IRB must first approve the study. IRBs are charged with ensuring that research is performed safely; with assessing the protection of human subjects and with making certain that each study meets institutional standards for scientific conduct. IRBs often also review adverse events. Importantly, this process has led to another area of concern, namely conflicts of interest in the composition of IRBs at academic medical centers and in the use of commercial or independent IRBs. Whereas the intent of the IRB is to harmonize the interests of clinical researchers with the protection of research subjects, the concern is that the IRB's primary function has apparently become the protection of the institution rather than the research subjects (Annas 1991). IRB membership is typically almost exclusively researchers from the particular institution, who therefore have a vested interest in the ongoing success of the institution. As Leslie Francis states the concern: members of the IRB may have "interests in job security; interests in the prestige or research reputation of the institution in which the IRB is located; commitments to scientific colleagues or to the advancement of technological medicine" (1996: 422; see also Slater 2002). Moreover, grant applications may include overhead reimbursements, payments for patient care, and so forth, which for a non-profit academic institution may be important sources of income. Similarly, members may be interested in the overall financial status of the for-profit or not-for-profit entity. The IRB is likely aware that the success of particular protocols may attract other profitable studies to the institution. Members may be friends, mentors, or colleagues of the investigators. At times, IRB members may informally coach the primary investigators on a research project regarding how best to phrase the protocol so that it will be approved. Also, members may bring a particular social, political, or moral agenda with them to the IRB; for example, they may be in favor of unfettered access to abortion or to unrestricted research on embryonic stem cells, and thus be more likely to approve even poorly designed studies that support such moral claims.

Similarly, insofar as certain research protocols or scientific theories are seen as supportive of particular political ideologies or sociopolitical movements, this may provide sufficient reason for some to fund, given credence to, or politically to support such research. Consider the ways in which human immunodeficiency virus (HIV)/ acquired immunodeficiency syndrome (AIDS) research has been highly politicized. When AIDS was identified in 1981 the homosexual community was deeply engaged in identity politics; that is, seeking tangible political goals, such as social acceptance, while elaborating an affirmative group identity (Epstein 1996: 11; Solvenko 1980). Such social and political concerns influenced the structure and goals of HIV/AIDS research. Criticizing mainstream scientific research as too slow, as antigay, and as failing to seek causes that were not associated with HIV transmission through sexual behavior, activists demanded further governmentally supported scientific investigation (Epstein 1996: 8–9). Public speculation existed regarding whether drug trials for potential therapeutic agents would have been handled differently if the patients had been dying of advanced cancer with no known therapeutic agent (Rothman and Edgar 1992: 204). Activists engaged in research established back-ground knowledge about treatments, occasionally conducted their own drug trials, and declared themselves experts to speak on these issues. Moreover, they claimed the expertise to define public health constructs, such as the practices that constituted "safe sex" (Epstein 1996: 8–9), challenged the linkage between sexual promiscuity and death, and put forward "sex positive" programs of AIDS prevention, which asserted as a moral community, however diffuse, the rights to sexual pleasure and sexual freedom. In addition to the potential biases of expert members of IRBs, external lay members may bring a moral, social, or political agenda with them to IRB discussions.[14]

Possible solutions have included a national or central review board to provide oversight of the local review boards (Christian *et al.* 2002) and commercial indepen-dent review boards (Forster 2002; Lemmens and Freedman 2000). In each case, how-ever, the central challenges appear to be unaddressed. Since independent review boards are typically financed through fee-for-service review they face similar financial conflicts of interest vis-à-vis the institution that is paying for the review (see e.g. Barnes and Florencio 2002a,b; Cave and Holm 2002; Lemmens and Thompson 2001). Moreover, both central and independent review boards may bring a moral or political agenda to their review of protocols.

Consider also the publication of results. Many scientific journals require that researchers disclose their funding sources as part of the manuscript review process, although standards vary regarding the disclosure of such information with the publication of the article. Some, such as the *British Medical Journal*, disclose funding sources, whereas others, such as *Nature*, do not. Here the common view is that scientists should have easy access to the investigational data of scientific inquiry. Sponsors of every type of study have some agenda that might possibly affect study design or data interpretation and presentation. As a result, if journals suppress certain studies because of their funding sources then the scientific community may reach false or distorted conclusions when considering a body of research. Journals usually rely on the use of a body of experts in the field of study, who conduct blinded peer review, to sustain the practice of professional scientific investigation.

A related problem is the underreporting of negative findings. Insofar as early results are negative, researchers—whether in the academy or commercial industry—may simply halt the trials. If unsuccessful trials typically go unpublished, this may lead to an unbalanced set of information for other scientists and practicing physicians. Commentators have reported that studies funded by pharmaceutical companies are 8 times less likely to report unfavorable qualitative conclusions than nonprofit funded studies and 1.4 times more likely to reach positive qualitative conclusions (Friedberg *et al.* 1999). Such findings do not impeach the quality of the research but they do suggest the need for a larger body of evidence available for clinical researchers to explore. In response to such concerns, in September, 2004, the International Committee of Medical Journal Editors announced that their representative journals—including *The New England Journal of Medicine*, *The Lancet*, and *The Journal of the American Medical Association*—had established a policy that if a company hopes to publish the results of a clinical trial in these journals, it must register the trial in a public database before it begins. Investigators are required to describe the condition the trial aims to treat, the drug to be tested, and the methods for data interpretation, such as specification of the standards that will measure success or failure. The announced goal is to reduce the selective reporting of trials (DeAngelis *et al.* 2004). In response, the Pharmaceutical Research and Manufacturers Association (PhRMA) announced the creation of a public database to hold the results of all controlled clinical trials completed since October 2002 for its members' drug products approved in the United States (www.clinicalstudyresults.org).

Still, some organizations actively prohibit the publication of research with certain types of industry sponsorship. The American Thoracic Society, for example, will not publish research funded by the tobacco industry. Their public statement on manuscript submission states: "On the Manuscript Submission Form, authors must certify that no part of the research presented has been funded by tobacco industry sources" (American Thoracic Society 2004). Here, the challenge is to avoid policies that impede the progress of science in the search for untainted money, or that otherwise promotes a particular social, political, or ideological purity in scientific research. As one editorial noted in response to the American Thoracic Society's policy:

> The peer review system is designed to try and ensure that the conclusions of studies are supported by the evidence they contain, but peer review cannot guarantee the validity of studies. Studies must be published so that other researchers can make up their own minds on their quality. Because peer review cannot guarantee the validity of a study and because bias operates very subtly, many journals, including this one, print authors' funding sources alongside

papers. By doing so, the journals ensure that the ultimate peer reviewers, practising doctors, can use that information to make up their own minds on the validity and usefulness of a piece of research.

(Roberts and Smith 1996: 133)

A central question, though, remains: how far must one go to divert oneself from other interests to preserve the objectivity of research? Should one consider the current holdings of one's mutual funds? Should one accept governmental funds acquired through coercive taxation? If one utilizes governmental funding to conduct research on human embryos then all citizens are complicit in what many believe to be gravely evil. Commercial and industrial private funding sources possess the virtue of only utilizing those who choose to collaborate.

A changing research environment: financing innovation in the academy

Beginning in the 1980s the federal government recast policy to encourage relationships between the academy and industry. Central to these changes, the Bayh-Dole Act (P.L. 96–517, Patent and Trademark Act Amendments of 1980) created incentives to spur on research and to encourage technology transfer—such as pharmaceuticals and medical devices—from the university setting to the commercial sector. Some of its major provisions permitted universities to retain title to innovations developed under federally funded research programs; encouraged universities to collaborate with commercial industry to promote utilization of the inventions; expected universities to file patents on inventions, and to give licensing preference to small business. Universities were legally able to obtain patents and licenses as well as to negotiate with industrial partners for royalties and other fees. In exchange, private industry gained access to significant research talent.[15] The expectation was that the results of basic research would more easily shift from the laboratory and clinical settings to industry, which in turn would utilize the research for commercial products. The public would thereby reap more efficiently and effectively the benefits of basic research.

The Bayh-Dole Act permitted universities to combine federal monies with industry support and retain the exclusive license for patents resulting from the research. As a direct result, the act encouraged industry to support the academic research environment, because licensing agreements protected their investments and work product. The consequence: there has been significant increase in the pace of innovation in pharmaceuticals and medical devices. Before the Bayh-Dole Act, the number of applications from universities was approximately 250 per year; after enactment, in 1998, there were over 4,800 (Association of University Technology Managers (AUTM) 2000; Editorial 2000: 299); in 2002 there were over 7,741 (AUTM 2003: 21). These two distinct cultures—the academic and the industrial— began to develop closer ties (Steiner 1996: 458),[16] with a more significant percentage of research funding coming from the private sector.

In 2000, private industry devoted approximately $55–60 billion dollars to research and development, which represented more than twice that spent by the government. Licensing income for universities increased from approximately

$186 million in 1991 to approximately $735 million in 1997 (Barnes and Florencio 2002b: 526; see also Culliton 1981). In a survey of 219 university and academic institutions, the AUTM reported a 2002 licensing income of $1.337 billion (AUTM 2003: 28). Faculty researchers, and sometimes the academic medical centers themselves, are increasingly incorporating private start-up companies further to test and develop products based on the research conducted at the academic institution. Some 4,320 such start-up companies have been formed since 1980, with approximately 2,741 or 63.4 percent still operational (AUTM 2003: 32–33; see also Council on Governmental Relations 1999). A general observation of such innovation is that over time it has advanced health-care science and patient care through the development of innovative pharmaceuticals, medical devices, and medical techniques.

Whereas it is commonplace to comment that such research has become a lucrative enterprise, it would be shortsighted not to note that it has also played a crucial role in demonstrating that many treatments thought to be important parts of the standard of care were ineffective or at least less effective than new alternatives. Such innovation has increased longevity while decreasing morbidity. Capitalist systems, by rewarding innovation and those who succeed in the market, tend to increase the standard of living and the availability of goods and services, such as medicine. Here one might consider advancements in material well-being represented by increasing life expectancy and decreasing infant mortality in the industrial world.[17] Medical research requires the investment of capital, and while governments fund some innovation, there are limits to the governmental resources that can be devoted to basic science. Moreover, the market is likely the most efficient means for securing and productively directing such investment. The competitive stimulus to gain financial and professional rewards drives innovation; it possesses significant motivational force independent of a disinterested concern for civic duty and scientific curiosity. Such financial rewards stimulate innovation as well as finance research and development. In the United States, industry finances approximately 57 percent of biomedical research, with the National Institute of Health (NIH) funding approximately 36 percent and nonprofit organizers 7 percent (Senate Joint Economics Committee 2000: 9). According to the industry group PhRMA, it costs approximately 10–15 years and $800 million to bring a new drug to market (PhRMA 2004), and only approximately 3 in 10 drugs will be sufficiently profitable to recoup this research and development expense.

The US Senate Joint Economics Committee estimates that the direct and indirect costs of illness in the United States exceed $3 trillion annually (2000: i); as a consequence, effectively and efficiently treating illness also directly impacts productivity and the gross domestic product. In one statistical study that considered the aggregate impact of new pharmaceuticals on health-care costs, hospital and surgery indicators declined most for those illnesses that had the most significant increase in pharmaceuticals prescribed. The study demonstrated that increased prescriptions and innovative pharmaceuticals reduced hospital admissions, number of hospital days, and the number of surgical procedures. It concluded that on average a 1-dollar increase in pharmaceutical spending translated into a 3-dollar-and-65 cent reduction in overall health-care expenses (Lichtenberg 1996). Thus, while the pursuit of innovative pharmaceuticals and medical devices is an important key to decreasing morbidity costs and mortality risks, it also improves productivity and may reduce long-term health-care expenditures.

Moreover, commercial industry stepped up to fund university-based research as federal budget deficits decreased the amount of money available to universities and academic scientists. Competition for research dollars has become increasingly steep with academic medical centers no longer receiving the bulk of research dollars. Compounding difficulties, as Marcia Angell notes, reductions in reimbursements from Medicare and third-party insurance payers left academic medical centers financially strapped (2000). In a survey of research leaders, 9 out of 10 reported that the pressure to treat patients and insufficient revenue from such clinical work poses a moderate to large problem for clinical research (Campbell *et al.* 2001: 805). This perception was greater in academic medical centers located in markets with a high degree of managed care penetration. External funding from the private sector—for example, pharmaceutical companies and so forth—often helps to make up for such shortfalls, facilitating the academic missions of research, education, and clinical care (Angell 2000: 1517).

Conclusion and areas for further studies

How much of one's life must be disclosed to preserve scientific professionalism? In addition to financing sources and commercial entanglements, political, moral, and other epistemic and non-epistemic background commitments often play roles in surreptitious or unconscious distortion of scientific data to acquire research funding, advance one's social standing in the scientific community, or further particular sociopolitical goals. The protection of careers and the furtherance of other professional and social goals may at times take precedence over scientific accuracy (Bell 1992; O'Toole 1991). Indeed, it would be shortsighted to overlook the pervasive and subtly nuanced conflicts that desire for renown, professional advancement, and moral worldview represent (Shimm and Spece 1996).

While the literature has focused almost exclusively on financial ties with commercial industry, it is important to note that commercial markets are not the only source of profit-seeking behavior. Private nonprofit associations often expect that sponsored research protocols will yield results that are supportive of the organization's goals. For example, if one is a recipient of a grant from the American Thoracic Society or the American Lung Association, insofar as one seeks grant renewal one might be hesitant to publish results that confirm health benefits attributable to cigarette smoking. There exists, for example, significant evidence that the nicotine in tobacco smoke assists in the prevention and treatment of active ulcerative colitis (Bristwistle and Hall 1996; Pullan *et al.* 1994; Sandborn *et al.* 1997), Parkinsonism and Alzheimer's disease (Gray *et al.* 1996), and it has been linked to the recovery of immune response that had been previously suppressed by immobilization stress (Gomita *et al.* 1996). Cigarette smoking has also been shown to heighten short-term and long-term learning ability, enhance one's ability to reason under stress and, more generally, to cope with stress (Fletcher 1988; Folkman and Lazarus 1991). In some areas, reporting such research might be seen as politically incorrect or morally unpopular.

Given the impact of such social and political prior commitments on the interpretation and significance of scientific findings, as well as on the structure and goals of science, governmentally supported, rather than market-based, medical research is no guarantee of truth-seeking behavior.[18] Further study regarding the impact of researchers' religious background, or lack of personal religious belief, political viewpoints, voting habits, or social agendas should be fruitful for understanding the ways in which such background worldviews subtly affect or unconsciously distort the way that one designs studies, collects, and interprets data.

Notes

1 As the American Medical Association Council on Ethical and Judicial Affairs states the issue:

> Under no circumstances may physicians place their own financial interests above the welfare of their patients. The primary objective of the medical profession is to render service to humanity; reward or financial gain is a subordinate consideration. For a physician to unnecessarily hospitalize a patient, prescribe a drug, or conduct diagnostic tests for the physician's financial benefit is unethical. If a conflict develops between the physician's financial interest and the physician's responsibilities to the patient, the conflict must be resolved to the patient's benefit.
>
> (2003: E 8.03)

2 *The Belmont Report* draws the distinction as follows:

> For the most part, the term "practice" refers to interventions that are designed solely to enhance the well-being of an individual patient or client and that have a reasonable expectation of success. The purpose of medical or behavioral practice is to provide diagnosis, preventive treatment or therapy to particular *individuals*. By contrast, the term "research" designates an activity designed to test an hypothesis, permit conclusions to be drawn, and thereby to develop or contribute to generalizable knowledge (expressed, for example, in theories, principles, and statements of relationships). Research is usually described in a formal protocol that sets forth an objective and a set of procedures designed to reach that objective.
>
> (National Commission 1979/2003: 127, section A)

3 Here the challenge is that the prevailing methodology of clinical trials includes a placebo arm in which patients do not receive potentially beneficial medication. The literature raises questions regarding whether such research is more efficient, effective, and statistically meaningful than trials using other drugs as active controls, better promotes medical science and patient welfare, or violates patient/physician trust. See, for example, Emanuel and Miller (2001), Freedman *et al.* (1996a,b), Lemmens and Miller (2002), Miller and Brody (2002).

4 Edmund Erde refers to moral judgments and sociopolitical goals broadly speaking as "ideals," that is,

> These are the values that provide a person with a sense of calling or meaning, and so should be thought of as intrinsic rather than instrumental. They may derive from religious or professional indoctrination or from independent decisions after reflection.
>
> (Erde 1996: 20)

5 George Khushf notes that it is easy to understand why the bulk of the literature on conflicts of interest focuses primarily on financial conflicts:

> This is an area where we find the most pervasive challenge to traditional professional obligations. New economic arrangements involve situations where the physician's financial self-interest is seen to diverge from the patient's medical interest, presumably leading to either the over or underutilization of services. Such commercial

arrangements are perceived as temptations in which the physician may violate classical fiduciary obligations to put the patient's interest above all else.

(1998: 114)

6 Here the claim is that there is an inducement actively to enroll patients who do not fully satisfy the study's criteria to obtain a sufficient number of subjects within the study's time-frame. Estimates regarding these payments range from $2,500 to $5,000, or perhaps even $6,000, per patient (Kaplan and Brownlee 1999; Roizen 1988; Shimm and Spece 1991). Per capita payments typically offset medical and data management expenses. However, insofar as payments exceed costs, there exist extra monies to fund other research opportunities, travel to scientific conferences, purchase office or laboratory equipment, or receive salary increases. Other types of per capita payments include financial incentives to boost patient enrollment, such as bonuses for meeting particular enrollment goals, or finder's fees for seeking out and enrolling appropriate subjects.

If researchers enroll patients who are inappropriate or only marginally appropriate for the study this may both impact the relevance of the study's data and harm patients. Subjects may thereby receive experimental drugs to treat medical conditions that they do not have. The case of Thomas Parham, discussed above, fits this profile. Or, subjects may be enrolled in a particular study when other treatments or research protocols are known to be more beneficial. Such choices may compromise patient care and undermine the trust between patient and physician (Lind 1990). Moreover, if the researcher is also the patient's physician there is the additional conflict of both needing to treat the patient and to obtain objective data. Some commentators have suggested that honestly documenting the method of research funding should be a required part of informed consent (Finkel 1991; Office of Inspector General 2000).

7 In part, the concern is that gifts may come with strings attached, such as prepublication review of any articles developed from data gleaned from use of the gift (Campbell *et al.* 1998). Corporate gifts may also affect a researcher's choice on the direction of research or to choose one protocol over another in hope of future gifts. Similarly, all-expense-paid trips to a vacation resort to participate in a seminar hosted by a pharmaceutical company may have an impact on one's research. For example, colleagues accused Dr Joseph Oesterling of failing accurately to report findings in a conference presentation regarding a study sponsored by ViaMed, which allegedly paid him thousands of dollars in honoraria and travel expenses. Dr Oesterling was a member of ViaMed's board of directors and owned 13,334 shares of its stock (Goldner 2000: 382). The general concern is that physicians, who are financially compensated, directly or indirectly by the company sponsoring the research, will be more likely to misrepresent the accuracy of test results, or less likely to report negative findings. The affect may not be outright fraud, but rather subtle, perhaps unintentional, shifts in an investigator's interpretation or presentation of data (Hilgartner 1990). One study found, for example, a statistically significant association between industry support and positive pro-industry conclusions (Bekelman *et al.* 2003; Friedman and Richter 2004). Such association was also associated with restrictions on publication and data sharing.

8 Here the concern is that industry support may be shifting research emphasis from basic research to clinical research in the hope of product development with more immediate commercial suitability (Blumenthal *et al.* 1986, 1996; Rabino 1998).

9 Lori B. Andrews reports that pharmaceutical companies at times pay physicians millions of dollars a year for enrolling patients in studies, with potentially poor results:

Doctors from one field enroll their patients in drug trials in another field. For example, asthma specialists run studies on psychiatric medications. Patients who are not appropriate candidates for a study have received drugs for conditions they did not have, sometimes without even being told that the drugs were experimental. That not only subjected them to unnecessary risks, which is malpractice, but also compromised the study results.

(Andrews 2000: B4)

10 Self-referral and physician ownership of clinical testing facilities raises additional concerns that, for the most part, go beyond the focus of this chapter. For an excellent study of these issues see Moore (2003), Stout and Warner (2003), and Zientek (2003).

11 Brody identifies eight possible sources of clinical trial design that can provide opportunity for those with a conflict of interest to promote a favored treatment. These included decisions regarding:

(1) Which treatments will be tested in the proposed trial, and which will not be tested?

(2) Will there be a placebo control group as well, or will the treatments be tested against each other or against some active control group?

(3) What will be taken as the favorable endpoint (the result constituting the evidence of the dangerousness of the treatment)?

(4) What will be the condition for inclusion or exclusion of subjects from the trial?

(5) What provisions will be made for informed consent?

(6) Under what conditions will the trial be stopped or modified because there have been too many adverse endpoints in one or more arms of the trial or because the preliminary data have shown that one of the treatments is clearly the most efficacious treatment?

(7) Under what conditions will the trial be stopped or modified because of the newly available results of other trials?

(8) Which patients who meet the criteria will actually be enrolled, and which ones will not?

(1996: 409)

Those with a conflict of interest might choose in ways, even if unconsciously, that lead to flaws in the study design rather than to flawed data.

12 The Association of American Universities' task force on conflict of interest adopted the following definition of individual conflict of interest:

The term conflict of interest in science refers to situations in which financial or other personal considerations may compromise, or have the appearance of compromising, an investigator's professional judgment in conducting or reporting research. The bias such conflicts may conceivably impart not only affects collection, analysis, and interpretation of data, but also the hiring of staff, procurement of materials, sharing of results, choice of protocol, involvement of human participants, and the use of statistical methods.

The task force determined that researchers were to disclose financial information that might pose a conflict of interest to the institution, to publications, in oral presentations, to federal agencies, and as part of the human participant review process.

(Hasselmo 2002: 424)

The task force also identified conflicts of interest at the institutional level, including university equity holdings, royalty arrangements, or licensing agreements, and the direction of research, as well as university officials who possess financial interests with industry partners. They offered the following definition:

An institutional financial conflict of interest may occur when the institution, any of its senior management or trustees, or a department, school, or other sub-unit, or a related organization (such as a university foundation) has an external relationship or financial interest in a company that itself has a financial interest in a faculty research project. Senior managers or trustees may also have conflicts when they serve on the boards of (or otherwise have an official relationship with) organizations that have significant commercial transactions with the university. The existence (or appearance) of such conflicts can lead to actual bias, or suspicion about possible bias, in the review or conduct of research at the university. If they are not evaluated or managed, they may result in choices or actions that are incongruent with the missions, obligations, or the values of the university.

13 Section §50.605 Management of conflicting interests, states that:

> The designated official(s) must: Review all financial disclosures; and determine whether a conflict of interest exists and, if so, determine what actions should be taken by the institution to manage, reduce, or eliminate such conflict of interest. A conflict of interest exists when the designated official(s) reasonably determines that a Significant Financial Interest could directly and significantly affect the design, conduct, or reporting of the PHS-funded research. Examples of conditions or restrictions that might be imposed to manage conflicts of interest include, but are not limited to:
>
> (1) Public disclosure of significant financial interests;
> (2) Monitoring of research by independent reviewers;
> (3) Modification of the research plan;
> (4) Disqualification from participation in all or a portion of the research funded by the PHS;
> (5) Divestiture of significant financial interests; or
> (6) Severance of relationships that create actual or potential conflicts.
>
> (ORI 2000)

14 According to Francis, lay members are most frequently clergy or lawyers. Moreover, they tend to have been appointed by high level institutional officials with whom they are associated, either through friendship or other official relationship (1996: 429).

15 "I see it as a two-way positive street. . . . Industry benefits because they get the best minds to help shape their research and also get the credibility that comes from having academics involved. Faculty benefit from industry relationships in that they get to have a voice in the cutting edge of what's going on in patient care and to shape the direction of research" (quoted in Boyd *et al.* 2003: 772).

16 Other researcher-industry ties are multifold. Marcia Angell summarizes:

> The ties between clinical researchers and industry include not only grant support, but also a host of other financial arrangements. Researchers serve as consultants to companies whose products they are studying, join advisory boards and speakers' bureaus, enter into patent and royalty arrangements, agree to be the listed authors of articles ghostwritten by interested companies, promote drugs and devices at company-sponsored symposiums, and allow themselves to be plied with expensive gifts and trips to luxurious settings. Many also have equity interest in the companies.
>
> (2000: 1516)

17 Consider the following changes in life expectancy at birth, comparing life expectancy in 1960 to life expectancy in 2002: United States: women: 73.1 versus 79.8 years; men: 66.6 versus 74.4; Turkey: women 50.3 versus 70.9; men: 46.3 versus 66.2; Greece: women 72.4 versus 80.7; men 67.3 versus 75.4; Mexico: women 59.2 versus 77.1; men 55.8 versus 72.1.

Also consider infant mortality per 1,000 live births, again comparing 1960 to 2002: United States: 26 versus 6.8; Turkey: 189.5 versus 38.3; Greece: 40.1 versus 5.9; Mexico: 79.3 versus 20.1.

18 One might also consider the Lysenko controversy in the former Soviet Union. T.D. Lysenko, a Soviet agronomist led an attack in the 1930s–1950s against classical genetics, arguing against both the gene concept and the theory of natural selection. He favored a vague Lamarckian notion of the inheritance of acquired characteristics, based in part on the principles of dialectical materialism. Both Stalin and later Khrushchev supported Lysenko. Critics were dismissed from their positions, their laboratories were closed, and at times were imprisoned. Researchers at times changed their scientific positions based on such non-epistemic political beliefs. Ernan McMullin cites the example of a geneticist Alikhanian who, at a session of the Lenin Academy of Agricultural Science in August of 1998, denounced the genetics he had formally taught arguing that the support of the

Central Committee of the Communist Party for Lysenko must be considered to be valid reason to regard his position as true (1987: 81; see also Joravsky 1970).

For an additional example, consider the way in which in the eighteenth and nineteenth centuries the moral offense of masturbation was transformed into a disease with somatic not just psychological dimensions. Chronic masturbation was considered a serious disorder leading to marked debility and occasionally death. It was held to be the cause of "dyspepsia, constrictions of the urethra, epilepsy, blindness, vertigo, loss of hearing, headache, impotency, loss of memory, 'irregular action of the heart', general loss of health and strength, rickets, leucorrhea in women, and chronic catarrhal conjunctivitis" (Engelhardt 1974: 236). The classification of masturbation as a disease incorporated moral assessments concerning deviancy, developed etiological accounts to explain and treat in a coherent fashion a manifold of displeasing signs and symptoms, and provided a direction for diagnosis, prognosis, and therapy. It thereby gave medical and conceptual structure to particular epistemic and non-epistemic values.

Bibliography

American Medical Association (AMA) Council on Ethical and Judicial Affairs (2003) *Code of Medical Ethics*, Chicago, IL: AMA.

American Thoracic Society (2004) "Manuscript Submission Form," Online available: http://www.thoracic.org/publications/ajrccm/bluecont2a.asp#ats3 (accessed September 10, 2004).

Andrews, L.B. (2000) "Money is Putting People at Risk in Biomedical Research," *Chronicle of Higher Education*, 46(27): B4. March 10.

Angell, M. (2000) "Is Academic Medicine for Sale?," *The New England Journal of Medicine*, 342(20): 1516–18.

Annas, G. (1991) "Ethics Committees: From Ethical Comfort to Ethical Cover," *Hastings Center Report* 21(3): 18–21.

Association of University Technology Managers (AUTM) (2003) *The AUTM Licensing Survey: FY 2002*. Online available: http://www.autm.net (accessed November 15, 2004).

——(2000) *The AUTM Licensing Survey: FY 1998*. Online available: http://www.autm.net (accessed November 15, 2004).

Barnes, M. and Florencio, P. (2002a) "Financial Conflicts of Interest in Human Subjects Research: The Problem of Institutional Conflicts," *Journal of Law, Medicine, and Ethics*, 30: 390–402.

——(2002b) "Investigator, IRB, and Institutional Financial Conflicts of Interest in Human-Subjects Research: Past, Present and Future," *Seton Hall Law Review*, 32: 525–61.

Bekelman, J., Li, Y., and Gross, C.P. (2003) "Scope and Impact of Financial Conflicts of Interest in Biomedical Research," *Journal of the American Medical Association*, 289(4): 454–65.

Bell, R. (1992) *Impure Science*, New York: John Wiley & Sons, Inc.

Blumenthal, D., Campbell, E.G., Causino, N., and Louis, K.S. (1996) "Participation of Life-Science Faculty in Research Relationships with Industry," *New England Journal of Medicine*, 335: 1734–39.

Blumenthal, D., Gluck, M., Louis, K.S., Stoto, M.A., and Wise, D. (1986) "University Industry Research Relationships in Biotechnology: Implications for the University," *Science*, 232(4756): 1361–66.

Boyd, E.A., Cho, M.K., and Bero, L. (2003) "Financial Conflict-of-Interest Policies in Clinical Research: Issues for Clinical Investigators," *Academic Medicine*, 78(8): 769–74.

Bristwistle, J. and Hall, K. (1996) "Does Nicotine Have Beneficial Effects in the Treatment of Certain Diseases?," *British Journal of Nursing*, 5(19): 1195–202.

Brody, B.A. (1996) "Conflicts of Interests and the Validity of Clinical Trials," in R.G. Spece, Jr, D.S. Shimm, and A. Buchanan (eds) *Conflicts of Interest in Clinical Practice and Research* (pp. 407–17). New York: Oxford University Press.

Campbell, E.G., Louis, K.S., and Blumenthal, D. (1998) "Looking a Gift Horse in the Mouth: Corporate Gifts Supporting Life Sciences Research," *Journal of the American Medical Association*, 279: 996–99.

Campbell, E.G., Weissman, J.S., May, E., and Blumenthal, D. (2001) "Status of Clinical Research in Academic Health Centers: Views from Research Leadership," *Journal of the American Medical Association*, 286(7): 800–06.

Cave, E. and Holm, S. (2002) "New Governance Arrangements for Research Ethics Committees: Is Facilitating Research Achieved at the Cost of Participants' Interest," *Journal of Medical Ethics*, 28: 318–21.

Cherry, M. and Engelhardt, H.T., Jr (2004) "Informed Consent in Texas: Theory and Practice," *The Journal of Medicine and Philosophy*, 29: 237–52.

Cho, M., Shohara, R., Schissel, A., and Rennie, D. (2000) "Policies on Faculty Conflicts of Interest at US Universities," *Journal of the American Medical Association*, 284(17): 2203–08.

Christian, M., Goldberg, J., Killen, J., Abrams, J., McCabe, M., Mauer, J., and Wittes, R. (2002) "A Central Institutional Review Board for Multi-Institutional Trials," *New England Journal of Medicine*, 346(18): 1405–08.

Council on Governmental Relations (1999) "The Bayh-Dole Act: A Guide to the Law and Implementing Regulations," Online available: www.ucop.edu/ott/bayh.html (accessed January 25, 2005).

Culliton, B.J. (1981) "Biomedical Research Enters the Marketplace," *New England Journal of Medicine*, 304: 1195–201.

DeAngelis, C.D., Drazen, J.M., Frizelle, F.A., Haug, C., Hoey, J., Horton, R., Kotzin, S., Laine, C., Marusic, A., Overbeke, A.J., Schroeder, T.V., and Van der Weyden, M.B. (2004) "Clinical Trial Registration: A Statement from the International Committee of Medical Journal Editors," *Journal of the American Medical Association*, 292(11): 1363–64.

Editorial (2000) "Financial Conflicts of Interest," *Nature Neuroscience*, 3(4): 299.

Emanuel, E. and Miller, F. (2001) "The Ethics of Placebo Controlled Trials—A Middle Ground," *New England Journal of Medicine*, 345(12): 915–19.

Engelhardt, H.T., Jr (1996) *Foundations of Bioethics*, New York: Oxford University Press.

——(1974) "The Disease of Masturbation: Values and the Concept of Disease," *Bulletin of the History of Medicine*, 48: 234–48.

Epstein, S. (1996) *Impure Science: AIDS, Activism, and the Politics of Knowledge*, Berkeley, CA: University of California Press.

Erde, E. (1996) "Conflicts of Interest in Medicine: A Philosophical and Ethical Morphology," in R.G. Spece, Jr, D.S. Shimm, and A. Buchanan (eds) *Conflicts of Interest in Clinical Practice and Research* (pp. 12–41). New York: Oxford University Press.

Finkel, M.J. (1991) "Should Informed Consent Include Information on How Research is Funded?," *Institutional Review Board*, 13(5): 1–3.

Fletcher, B. (1988) "The Epidemiology of Occupational Stress," in C.L. Cooper and R. Payne (eds) *Causes, Coping and Consequences of Stress at Work* (pp. 3–50). New York: John Wiley & Sons Ltd.

Folkman, S. and Lazarus, R. (1991) "Coping and Emotion," in A. Monat and R. Lazarus (eds) *Stress and Coping* (pp. 62–80). New York: Columbia University Press.

Forster, D. (2002) "New Directions in Human Subject Research: Looking Beyond the Academic Medical Center: Independent Review Boards," *Seton Hall Law Review*, 32: 513–23.

Francis, L. (1996) "IRBs and Conflicts of Interest," in R.G. Spece, Jr, D.S. Shimm, and A. Buchanan (eds) *Conflicts of Interest in Clinical Practice and Research* (pp. 418–36). New York: Oxford University Press.

Freedman, B., Glass, K.C., and Weijer, C. (1996a) "Placebo Orthodoxy in Clinical Research II: Ethical, Legal, and Regulatory Myths," *Journal of Law, Medicine & Ethics*, 24: 252–59.

Freedman, B., Weijer, C., and Glass, K.C. (1996b) "Placebo Orthodoxy in Clinical Research I: Empirical and Methodological Myths," *Journal of Law, Medicine & Ethics*, 24: 243–51.

Friedberg, M., Saffran, B., Stinson, T., Nelson, W., and Bennett, C. (1999) "Evaluation of Conflict of Interest in Economic Analyses of New Drugs Used on Oncology," *Journal of the American Medical Association*, 282(15): 1453–57.

Friedman, L. and Richter, E. (2004) "Relationship between Conflicts of Interest and Research Results," *Journal of General Internal Medicine*, 19(1): 51–56.

Goldner, J.A. (2000) "Dealing with Conflicts of Interest in Biomedical Research: IRB Oversight as the Next Best Solution to the Abolitionist Approach," *The Journal of Law, Medicine & Ethics*, 28(4): 379–404.

Gomita, Y., Furuno, K., Matsuka, N., Yao, K., Oishi, R., Nishibori, M., Saeki, K., Nagai, H., Koda, A., and Shimizu, Y. (1996) "Effects of Nicotine and Exposure to Cigarette Smoke on Suppression of Local Graft-Versus-Host Reaction Inducted by Immobilization Stress in Mice," *Methods and Findings in Experimental and Clinical Pharmacology*, 18(9): 573–77.

Gray, R., Rajan, A.S., Radcliffe, K.A., Yakehiro, M., and Dani, J.A. (1996) "Hippocampal Synaptic Transmission Enhanced by Low Concentrations of Nicotine," *Nature* 383: 713–16.

Hasselmo, N. (2002) "Individual and Institutional Conflict of Interest: Policy Review by Research Universities in the United States," *Science and Engineering Ethics*, 8(3): 421–27.

Hilgartner, S. (1990) "Research Fraud, Misconduct and the IRB," *Institutional Review Board*, 12(1): 1–4.

Joravsky, D. (1970) *The Lysenko Affair*, Cambridge, MA: Harvard University Press.

Kaplan, S. and Brownlee, S. (1999) "Dying for a Cure: Why Cancer Patients Often Turn to Risky Experimental Treatments—and Wind up Paying with Their Lives," *US News & World Report*, 11(October): 34.

Khushf, G. (1998) "A Radical Rupture in the Paradigm of Modern Medicine: Conflicts of Interest, Fiduciary Obligations, and the Scientific Ideal," *The Journal of Medicine and Philosophy*, 23(1): 98–122.

Lemmens, T. and Freedman, B. (2000) "Ethics Review for Sale? Conflict of Interest and Commercial Research Review Boards," *Milbank Quarterly*, 78(4): 547–83.

Lemmens, T. and Miller, P. (2002) "Avoiding a Jekyll-and-Hyde Approach to Ethics of Clinical Research and Practice," *American Journal of Bioethics*, 2(2): 14–17.

Lemmens, T. and Thompson, A. (2001) "Noninstitutional Commercial Review Boards in North America," *IRB: Ethics and Human Research*, 23(2): 1–12.

Lichtenberg, F.R. (1996) "The Effect of Pharmaceutical Utilization and Innovation on Hospitalization and Mortality," National Bureau of Economic Research Working Paper 5418.

Lind, S.L. (1990) "Finder's Fees for Research Subjects," *New England Journal of Medicine*, 323: 192–95.

Lo, B., Wolf, L., and Berkeley, A. (2000) "Conflict-of-Interest Policies for Investigators in Clinical Trials," *The New England Journal of Medicine*, 343(22): 1616–20.

McMullin, E. (1987) "Scientific Controversy and Its Termination," in H.T. Engelhardt, Jr and A. Caplan (eds) *Scientific Controversies* (pp. 49–92). Cambridge: Cambridge University Press.

Medical Research Council (2003) "Good Research Practice," in S. Eckstein (ed.) *Manual for Research Ethics Committees*, 6th edn (pp. 207–13). Cambridge: Cambridge University Press.

Miller, F.G. and Brody, H. (2002) "What Makes Placebo-Controlled Trials Unethical?," *American Journal of Bioethics*, 2(2): 3–9.

Moore, N.J. (2003) "Regulating Self-Referrals and Other Physician Conflicts of Interest," *Health Care Ethics Committee Forum*, 15(2): 134–54.

National Commission for the Protection of Human Subjects of Biomedical and Behavioral Research (1979/2003) "The Belmont Report: Ethical Principles and Guidelines for the Protection of Human Subjects of Research," in S. Eckstein (ed.) *Manual for Research Ethics Committees*, 6th edn (pp. 126–32). Cambridge: Cambridge University Press.

Office of Inspector General (2000) "Recruiting Human Subjects: Pressures in Industry Sponsored Clinical Research," Washington, DC: Office of Inspector General, Department of Health and Human Services.

Office of Research Integrity (ORI) (2000) "Responsibility of Applicants for Promoting Objectivity in Research for which PHS Funding is Sought," 42 CFR 50.601–07.

Organization for Economic Co-operation and Development (2004) *Health Data 2004*, 1st edn, Table 1: Life Expectancy (in years); Table 2: Infant Mortality, Deaths per 1000 Live Births. Online available: www.oecd.org (accessed January 25, 2005).

O'Toole, M. (1991) "Margot O'Toole's Record of Events," *Nature*, 351: 183.

PhRMA (2004) "The Issues: Intellectual Property," Online available: www.pharma.org (accessed June 24, 2004).

Pullan, R.D., Rhodes, J., Ganesh, S., Mani, V., Morris, J.S., Williams, G.T., Newcombe, R.G., Russell, M., Feyerabend, C., Thomas, G., and Sawe, U. (1994) "Transdermal Nicotine for Active Ulcerative Colitis," *New England Journal of Medicine*, 330: 811–15.

Rabino, I. (1998) "Societal and Commercial Issues Affecting the Future of Biotechnology in the United States: A Survey of Researchers' Perceptions," *Naturwissenschaften*, 85: 109–16.

Roberts, J. and Smith, R. (1996) "Publishing Research Supported by the Tobacco Industry," *British Medical Journal*, 312: 133–34.

Roizen, R. (1988) "Why I Oppose Drug Company Payment of Physician/Investigators on a Per Patient/Subject Basis," *Institutional Review Board*, 10(1): 9–10.

Rothman, D. and Edgar, H. (1992) "Scientific Rigor and Medical Realities: Placebo Trials in Cancer and AIDS Research," in E. Fee and D. Fox (eds) *AIDS: The Making of a Chronic Disease* (pp. 194–206). Berkeley, CA: University of California Press.

Sandborn, W.J., Tremaine, W.J., Offord, K.P., Lawson, G.M., Peterson, B.T., Batts, K.P., Croghan, I.T., Dale, L.C., Schroeder, D.R., and Hurt, R.D. (1997) "Transdermal Nicotine for Mildly to Moderately Active Ulcerative Colitis; A Randomized, Double Blind, Placebo-Controlled Trial," *Annals of Internal Medicine*, 126(5): 364–71.

Senate Joint Economics Committee (2000) *The Benefits of Medical Research and the Role of the NIH*, May, Washington, DC: US Senate.

Shimm, D.S. and Spece, R.G., Jr (1996) "An Introduction to Conflicts of Interest in Clinical Research," in R.G. Spece, Jr, D.S. Shimm, and A. Buchanan (eds) *Conflicts of Interest in Clinical Practice and Research* (pp. 361–75). New York: Oxford University Press.

——(1991) "Conflict of Interest and Informed Consent in Industry-Sponsored Clinical Trials," *Journal of Legal Medicine*, 12: 477–513.

Slater, E.E. (2002) "IRB Reform," *New England Journal of Medicine*, 346(18): 1402–04.

Solvenko, R. (1980) "Homosexuality and the Law: From Condemnation to Celebration," in J. Marmor (ed.) *Homosexual Behavior: A Modern Reappraisal*. New York: Basic Books.

Steiner, D. (1996) "Competing Interests: The Need to Control Conflict of Interest in Biomedical Research," *Science and Engineering Ethics*, 2(4): 457–68.

Stout, S. and Warner, D. (2003) "How Did Physician Ownership Become a Federal Case? The Stark Amendments and Their Prospects," *Health Care Ethics Committee Forum*, 15(2): 171–87.

Thompson, D.F. (1993) "Understanding Financial Conflicts of Interest," *The New England Journal of Medicine*, 329(8): 573–76.

Zientek, D. (2003) "Physician Entrepreneurs, Self-Referral, and Conflicts of Interest: An Overview," *Health Care Ethics Committee Forum*, 15(2): 111–33.

10 Interpreting scientific data ethically

A frontier for research ethics

Griffin Trotter

On January 30, 1997, CBS Evening News did a segment on the use of thrombolytics ("clot busters") in acute stroke. The story was spun as yet another instance of uninformed doctors and patients failing to avail themselves of the latest and best scientific treatments. Dan Rather was indignant:

> When it comes to treatment for stroke, study after study has shown that drugs called "clot busters" can limit, sometimes even reverse the crippling effects and brain damage, but only if they're given in time. So why are the vast majority of stroke patients not being treated with them?
>
> (Rather 1997)

The answer to Dan Rather's pointed question is very easy. Most acute stroke patients were not being treated with thrombolytics because (1) the vast majority of acute stroke patients were not eligible to receive them according to guidelines used in the National Institute for Neurological Disorders and Stroke (NINDS) trial and recapitulated by the American Heart Association (AHA) and other professional groups, and (2) even for seemingly eligible patients, there were (and still are) good reasons for withholding the drug in most clinical settings. Rather tells us that "study after study" demonstrated the effectiveness of thrombolytics. But actually, at this telling, only 1 of 5 randomized controlled clinical trials (RCTs) on thrombolytics in acute stroke had yielded positive results. Three others had been discontinued because of excess mortality in the group receiving thrombolytics (Donnan *et al.* 1996; Multicenter Acute Stroke Trial 1995, 1996). In a fourth, the study reached completion, but with an increased mortality of 50 percent in the patients who received thrombolytics (Hacke *et al.* 1995). The only positive trial—the NINDS trial—was a small study (624 patients) that showed modest functional gains with no mortality benefit (NINDS 1995). Even if the results of the NINDS trial could be reproduced in community hospitals (a dubious proposition), most stroke patients would not be eligible to receive the drug and only 1 in 9 of those who did get it would be expected to benefit (while perhaps 1 or more in 16 would suffer major complications) (Caplan 1997; Katzan *et al.* 2000). Overall, benefits to be derived from thrombolytics are relatively insignificant from a public health standpoint (Jorgensen *et al.* 1999)—especially in comparison to those obtainable by correcting hyperlipidemia, hypertension, inactivity, tobacco use, and other major risk factors for cerebrovascular disease. Worst of all—at least from the standpoint of bioethics' principle of nonmaleficence—implementation of thrombolytic protocols for stroke would mean that some patients with relatively benign afflictions such as transient ischemic attacks (TIAs) and atypical migraine syndromes would be mistakenly diagnosed with acute ischemic stroke, treated with thrombolytics, and killed by thrombolytics' most worrisome side effect: brain hemorrhage.

So why were thrombolytics for acute stroke considered to be such an important breakthrough and fabulous news story? Part of the answer is brisk marketing—not merely from Genentech (manufacturer of the thrombolytic tissue plasminogen activator (tPA)), but also from medical researchers and specialists. On the basis of the NINDS study, professional organizations rapidly formulated guidelines advocating the use of thrombolytics in acute stroke and declared "consensus" about its use. Physician experts lauded thrombolytics with the greatest hyperbole—declaring "the decade of the brain," "a new era of proactive rather than reactive stroke therapy," and "a milestone in the transformation of stroke from a realm of fatalism to a field of therapeutic opportunities." Some experts misleadingly implied not only that thrombolytic stroke therapy would have a major impact, but even that it would save many lives (despite the absence of evidence that it saves lives at all).[1] The falsehood about saving lives was rapidly assimilated by the media—perhaps largely because salvation came so rapidly and (they fancied) so dramatically.[2] One of the most distressing results of all this activity is that RCTs of thrombolytics in acute stroke stopped abruptly—despite important unresolved issues (such as their effectiveness in small community hospital settings) and an overall paucity of data. Once medical authorities pronounced their consensus about the beneficial effects of tPA in acute stroke, another RCT seemed superfluous.

If there is an appropriate object of indignation in the thrombolytics-for-stroke affair, it is media pundits such as Dan Rather and the medical experts who exhibited a strong pro-treatment bias in their interpretation of the scientific data—not the doctors they chided for withholding thrombolytics. Yet the ethical problem resides not so much with these or any particular individuals, but rather with faulty mechanisms and procedures by which scientific data are interpreted for professionals, administrators, policy makers, news media, and the general public. This affair and many others like it point to a vacuum in the corpus on research ethics—namely, the relative absence of inquiry into the ethics of interpreting scientific data once it has been produced. This essay attempts to help initiate such inquiry by considering four overlapping questions related to the ethical interpretation of scientific data: (1) Which scientific data warrant our attention? (2) Who should we trust to analyze this data? (3) How should data be interpreted to clinicians, other professionals, and regulators? and (4) How should data be interpreted to the general public? Because these questions are closely related, much of the discussion in any particular section of this chapter will be relevant to some of the others.

There are, of course, other interesting questions related to the ethical interpretation of data. For example, when should scientific data be withheld from the public?[3] and when is scientific data sufficient to warrant changes in the legal standard of care?[4] But the earlier four questions constitute a center of gravity for a relatively new and important realm of inquiry in research ethics.[5] I will deal with each of these only briefly and suggestively, citing the thrombolytic affair and the US Department of

Agriculture (USDA) nutritional guidelines for illustration. Most of the hard work remains for others. Though I have focused on scientific data pertaining to biomedicine, much of what I say is likely to apply to the practical interpretation of scientific data from other domains.

Before I commence, it may be worthwhile to note that this chapter is *not* about the ethics of evidence-based-medicine (EBM). EBM focuses on clinicians' decision-making and (in distinction to this essay) is not primarily concerned with the initial interpretation of scientific data and how it is communicated to professionals, news media, and the public. The ethics of EBM is an important domain of inquiry that has already begun to receive attention (Goodman 2003; Mills and Spencer 2003).

First question: which scientific data warrant our attention?

Ideally, all scientific data would be carefully reviewed for methodological soundness and clinical relevance. Adequately rigorous studies then would be interpreted for a wider audience and, where applicable, vigorously debated.

That is not what happens. Currently business, political, journalistic, and cultural factors affect which scientific data will be briskly interpreted. If manufacturers have robust profits at stake, if prominent researchers have invested great amounts of time and effort, if data pertain to hypotheses that yield potentially radical conceptual or practical shifts (especially the promise of something to do when hitherto clinicians could only stand around), or if studies are favored by politically powerful interest groups, then positive results are apt to be widely trumpeted and equivocal results likely to receive a positive spin, then great publicity. Conversely, if no fortunes, careers or therapeutic revolutions are at stake, attention will be predictably sparse (or absent); if negative results actually threaten profits or careers, they may be suppressed.

Part of the problem resides outside our focus—in values that initiate research. Most basic clinical research in the United States is funded by the federal government (Frist 2002). Most clinical drug trials are funded by pharmaceutical and device manufacturers (Bodenheimer 2000).[6] Much of the rest is funded by wealthy, disease-specific advocacy groups. Each of these sources introduces substantial bias—political, economic, and cultural—into what we choose to study (I'll call this "initiation bias," though I have not seen this term in use). Political and cultural influences have long dictated, for instance, that breast cancer studies receive more funding than lung cancer studies—even though lung cancer kills more women than breast cancer does.[7] Economic forces beget oodles of pills for erectile dysfunction, while two of the world's most lethal scourges—tuberculosis and malaria—have virtually no remedies in the pharmaceutical pipeline.

More germane to our specific question is the widely acknowledged problem of "publication bias"—an overly optimistic interpretation resulting when positive studies get published and discussed while negative or equivocal studies do not (Stern and Simes 1998). There is evidence, for instance, that many reviewers favor studies with statistically significant findings (Misakian and Bero 1998). Recently scholars and journal editors have strived to evaluate and reform the peer-review process[8] and eliminate conflicts of interest and other sources of bias (Baltic 2001; Cantekin *et al.* 1990; Horrobin 1990).

The problem of publication bias is exacerbated when drug manufacturers suppress unwanted data. Though members of the Pharmaceutical Research and Manufacturers of America (PhRMA) recently pledged to release all "meaningful study results, regardless of outcome," the enactment of this measure has been questioned. For instance, in June 2004, New York State Attorney General Eliot Spitzer sued British drug maker GlaxoSmithKline PLC for fraudulently withholding studies suggesting that one of its antidepressants was ineffective for children and adolescents, and might lead individuals in this age range to suicide.[9]

Initiation bias, publication bias, and drug companies' suppression of unfavorable data are refractory problems at best, but at least they are being addressed. An equally challenging but less publicized problem is the manner in which society deals with readily available data. Most consumers of medical data have neither the time nor the inclination to go directly to its sources. They receive much of their information passively, after it is carefully screened by drug companies, news media, or various experts. Doctors receive considerable information from pharmaceutical representatives who carefully choose which studies they will present (Wazana 2000). Even food makers have started marketing favored data directly to physicians.[10] News media are also choosy—often opting for drama (e.g., studies about clot busters) over practical relevance (e.g., studies about the effects of a sensible diet).

Some of the solutions are straightforward. Physicians need to get drug representatives out of the office. News media need to examine their typical "beat" sources for objectivity, and augment their reliance on press releases from politically engaged organizations such as the AHA, the American Medical Association (AMA), the National Stroke Association, and so forth, with input from more rigorously neutral sources.[11]

How will we replace the mainstays of information sorting? A good first step is turning to independent review organizations. In emergency medicine (my own particular clinical specialty), Emergency Medical Abstract (EMA) is one of several such sources. Every month, EMA analysts review hundreds or thousands of articles from hundreds of journals, then select about forty of the best, for which they write abstracts which are added to the subscriber's database. They also tape a session in which two analysts discuss the scientific merit and the clinical applicability of the selected studies. Their reviews are erudite and conspicuously unaffected by medicine's orthodox power structures (EMA is beholden only to subscribers). Well-educated members of the news media could subscribe to EMA and similar offerings—or develop their own specific sources of scientific input that exhibit comparable high standards.

Second question: whom should we trust to analyze scientific data?

The EMA example brings us to our second question. It is perhaps even more important to analyze scientific data appropriately than it is to be adept at choosing the right scientific data to analyze. After all, a good analysis of the wrong data exhibits the fact that it is not good or useful data, and that will stimulate a hunt for better or more relevant data.

The primary problem in current practice is that the first and much of the subsequent publicly marketed interpretation of scientific data is ordinarily provided by researchers who generate the data and colleagues with a similar stake in promoting it (Choudry *et al.* 2002). It would be difficult to select more biased sources (Chan *et al.* 2004). Aside from obvious and well-publicized financial incentives to spin their data positively (DeAngelis *et al.* 2001), most researchers exhibit several characteristics that potentially beget bias. In the context of the conduct of research most of these characteristics are virtues. But for interpreters they are liabilities.

First is the natural and laudable tendency of researchers to believe fervently in the importance of their subject matter. This tendency is amplified in two ways: (1) Researchers are prone to "preoccupation bias"—or what philosopher John Dewey called the "fallacy of selective emphasis" (Dewey 1988)—occurring when thinkers unintentionally but systematically exaggerate the importance of a particular point of interest because they are preoccupied with studying it. (2) Even apart from particular investigations, researchers presumably choose their specialties and life projects in much the same manner as other people who have the luxury of choice—by selecting a domain that interests them intensely and seems important. In their work, they are surrounded by many others who share this perspective. This commendable quality goes awry when researchers or groups of professionals seize the opportunity to convert their devotions into public policy. Perhaps the most brazen example is the World Health Organization's definition of health—in which they anoint themselves as high authority on everything that really matters for human fulfillment (Callahan 1990). But less grandiose examples, such as neurologists' fervent advocacy for thrombolytics in acute stroke vis-à-vis their relative complacence about more important preventive measures, also make an impact.

Second, researchers are naturally loyal to individuals and organizations who support their efforts (financially, intellectually, and otherwise), and want to reward this support with positive results. Only a cynic could relegate this loyalty to crass financial self-interest. To the contrary, loyalty should be regarded as a moral requirement for good researchers. Ideally, loyalty would be directed primarily toward high investigative standards, public benefit, and the search for truth.[12] But clinical studies are initiated because there is an expectation that they will yield fruitful results. This stimulus will always threaten the objectivity of researchers, even the best and most objective ones.

Third, researchers work in a competitive environment. Success in publications and in procuring research support is a prerequisite for advancement. Financial incentives certainly enter here. But professional self-esteem and a sense of accomplishment are perhaps greater incentives. Professional life is enhanced for researchers on nearly every front when studies prove to be noteworthy, important, and well executed. We should hardly expect them to be totally honest (even to themselves) about all of the ways in which their work does not exhibit these qualities.

McCormack and Greenhalgh have recognized the bias that results when researchers interpret their own data, and suggest that journal editors "encourage authors to present their results initially with a minimum of discussion so as to invite a range of comments and perspectives from readers" (McCormack and Greenhalgh 2000). Following their lead, I suggested in 2002 that journal editors turn to a cadre of experienced, neutral interpreters with special methodological expertise, and offered two strategies (Trotter 2002a). First, medical centers and universities could distinguish between two types of faculty appointment: clinician-researcher and clinician-interpreter. Clinician-researchers would continue to be mostly superspecialists (medical sub-specialists with expertise in study design and focused interests that occupy most of their clinical and research time) with appropriate ties to government, industry, and private funding organizations. Clinician-interpreters, on the other hand, would tend to be generalists with special training in interpreting clinical data who would eschew entrepreneurial ties. Second, medical journals, medical societies, and government regulators could assemble boards of expert clinician-interpreters to review studies and interpret their significance. This policy would be a significant departure from current practices—where researchers elaborate long "discussion" sections in the initial publication of their studies, and where medical societies and government regulators tend to commission panels of heavily invested expert researchers (often composed entirely of those who have published studies pertaining to the topic of interest). A consensus among such biased sources may not be the best standard of interpretive quality.

Third question: how should scientific data be interpreted to clinicians, other professionals, and regulators?

The current reliance on "consensus panels" is problematic in the interpretation of scientific data for two reasons: (1) as mentioned earlier, these panels are often composed of a select group of interpreters with group-specific biases, and (2) the quest for consensus tends to result in suppression of legitimate conflicts that should be highlighted. Both of these liabilities are apparent in initial recommendations about the use of thrombolytics in acute stroke.

When the Peripheral and Central Nervous System Drugs Advisory Committee of the Food and Drugs Administration (FDA) considered the use of tPA for acute stroke, the testimony came largely from clinical investigators involved in the NINDS trial. Most of these persons were also employed by Genentech, the company that markets tPA. The Advisory Committee itself was skewed—consisting entirely of neurologic specialists without a single emergency physician or radiologist (despite the fact that these latter specialties would be intimately involved in the use of thrombolytics for acute stroke) (Peripheral and Central Nervous System Drugs Advisory Committee 1996). Though public participation was invited, the only person to speak up was Karen Putney, a representative from the National Stroke Association (NSA). Her testimony is instructive:

> NSA understands that finding a treatment for acute ischemic stroke for which there is yet no approved therapy will do more than anything else to improve public awareness and understanding, compel the medical community to treat stroke emergently, and improve patient outcomes. This study heralds a new approach to stroke and carries the hope of transforming the hopelessness surrounding stroke into active, aggressive, and effective intervention to salvage brain tissue, reduce disability, and save lives.
>
> (Peripheral and Central Nervous System
> Drugs Advisory Committee 1996)

This brief statement exemplifies many of the false dogmas about thrombolytics for acute stroke: (1) that it saves lives, (2) that it constitutes a well-supported and important revolution in stroke therapy, and most distressingly, (3) that it ought to be converted into the standard of care, such that ordinary clinicians are compelled (presumably by threat of tort) to use it. Among the FDA's panel of neurological specialists, it was well received, and tPA was approved for the treatment of acute stroke despite a total absence of evidence for the external validity of the NINDS protocol applied to community hospitals and other sites with less experience, expertise, and equipment than researchers employed in the NINDS trial.[13]

After FDA approval, the bandwagon quickly grew larger. The AHA was one of several organizations that convened a consensus conference to produce guidelines for the use of thrombolytics in acute stroke. They recruited an emergency physician— Jerome R. Hoffman—for the conference, but dropped his name from their list of panel members when he refused to sign the resulting recommendations (with which he disagreed) (Hoffman 2001). Though Hoffman was invited to submit a rebuttal essay, this submission was never published. Later, Hoffman asked if the AHA would publish a shorter one- to two-paragraph dissent alongside the recommendations. When AHA refused, he asked that the following statement be appended to the document: "Jerome R. Hoffman also participated in the panel but disagrees with the recommendations contained in this paper." This request was also denied.

Ethical issues arising from such attempts at railroading a "consensus" are evident. Though bioethicists have investigated the notion of consensus and how it applies in their discipline (Trotter 2002b), more work is needed on ethical uses and abuses of scientific consensus. It is important that legitimate scientific controversies (controversies hinging on differing models of pathophysiology, therapeutics, etc.; but *not* controversies hinging on diverging economic objectives) be allowed to work themselves out without preemption. As Jonathan Moreno has observed, "one often has the feeling that, once consensus is announced by the appropriate individual or group, permission is implicitly given for mentation on the matter to cease" (Moreno 1995). When groups such as the AHA, AMA, American College of Emergency Physicians, and so forth circulate diagnostic and treatment standards, the momentum for challenge and dissent typically wanes.

Perhaps scientific consensus panels would do better if they employed clinician-interpreters of the sort discussed in the last section. In any case, some sort of account is needed of procedures that should be followed and results obtained before someone can validly announce a consensus of scientific experts.

Fourth question: how should data be interpreted to the general public?

A good illustration of pitfalls in the interpretation of scientific data for the general public is the construction of dietary guidelines and the food pyramid by the USDA. The guidelines provide a basis for all federal nutrition programs, including the school lunch program, and the pyramid is widely circulated for instructional purposes to the public. They are revised every five years in order to reflect the most recent scientific data. But the process is hardly driven by an unbiased assessment of scientific data.

The first step is the selection of thirteen experts to serve on the guidelines panel (the reconstruction of the pyramid is subsequently done by the USDA behind closed doors). As Leila Abboud of the *Wall Street Journal* reports, many industry groups know in advance what the experts' opinions will be, because "many of the nutrition researchers are affiliated with them, serving on their boards, doing research, and taking on speaking engagements" (Abboud 2003). Groups such as the National Dairy Council and the United Fresh Fruit and Vegetable Association submit names of favored candidates.

Then comes the wrangling. In 1995, experts sponsored by alcohol groups managed to get the committee to include the following line: "Alcoholic beverages have been used to enhance the enjoyment of meals by many societies throughout human history." However, under pressure from candidates recommended by advocacy groups such as the Center for Science in the Public Interest, this sentence was dropped in 2000. Abboud reports that the Sugar Association fought hard against the 2000 panel recommendation to "choose beverages and foods that limit your intake of sugars," and got it changed to "moderate your intake of sugars." Likewise, a representative of the Soft Drink Association has vowed to "counter allegations from the activist community, and public misperceptions that there is evidence to link sugar and obesity" (Abboud 2003).

It is troubling that taxpayer money is being utilized to fund such ineffective efforts to inform and guide the public. Other sources of public information do not fare much better. Direct-to-consumer drug marketing, for instance, permeates the airwaves with propaganda dressed up to look like scientific information.[14] And news media frequently convert data into meaningless sound and print bytes. Yet, though I have been critical of the media, it seems much more workable (and desirable) to improve news media performance than to try to eliminate their role and substitute other sources. Already, citizens are far too reliant on expensive sources of information (such as doctors' visits), or bad sources (such as USDA panels) for problems and issues that could be handled quickly and inexpensively through recourse to a savvy news media (including Internet sources). A sophisticated news media seems potentially the best source of scientific information for the general public. To transform itself, it will have to scrutinize its emphasis on dramatic narratives, preposterous claims, interpersonal conflicts, and anything sexy (Evans 1999). Somehow, the entertainment function must be more clearly differentiated from the informational function—a prospect that seems more likely in the print media (where balanced, informative, and useful reporting is already frequently evident). In a free country, we will always have biased, bombastic reporting. But increasingly sophisticated and involved health-care consumers will reward efforts to disseminate information in a less-biased manner.

Conclusion

Given the current explosion of research in medicine and other practical sciences, it is evident that clinicians, hospital administrators, policy makers, and lay persons will become increasingly dependent on others to interpret data for them. Interpretation can be accomplished well or poorly, ethically or unethically.

The ethics of interpreting scientific data considers data availability and worthiness of data for detailed interpretation, proper sources of interpretation, and proper procedures for interpretation. Sources and procedures for interpreting data for professionals and persons with sophisticated knowledge will differ from sources and procedures for interpreting data for the general public. In the former case, scientific journals, professional associations, and regulatory bodies bear much of the burden. Lay persons, on the other hand, will rely on media sources including the Internet (except when they receive information directly from professionals such as treating physicians).

As a stimulus to inquiry, we have examined a few instances where the interpretation of scientific data has been poorly executed. These examples (e.g., thrombolytics for acute stroke; federal nutritional guidelines) are of course just the tip of the iceberg. Yet we have discovered several general sources of ethical concern that warrant further analysis. These include (1) suppression of relevant data by moneyed interests, (2) the employment of biased researchers to interpret data for medical journals, policy makers, and the news media, (3) the emphasis among news media on entertainment value over reliable, unbiased interpretation, and (4) pressure to announce consensus when there are good reasons for airing critical dissent.

Notes

1 For example, Landis *et al.* 1997 wrote: "With the tools in hand, recognition of ischemic stroke as a medical emergency and application of prudent thrombolytic techniques will have a major impact on stroke morbidity and mortality."

2 US News and World Report (Schrof 1999) featured the following narrative:

> One Wednesday evening in January, 36-year-old Laurie Lucas was rushing about, dressing her daughters for school and talking on the phone, when a strange confusion swept over her. She felt woozy. Her right arm flailed about and her right leg went weak. Paramedics arriving at Lucas's Sanford, Fla., home thought she was having epileptic seizures, but brain scans revealed a blockage of an artery that supplies the brain with blood. Lucas, a physically fit former professional cheerleader, had suffered a massive stroke.
>
> If Lucas had been stricken a year ago, before a new treatment was developed, she almost certainly would have died. In fact, until recently there was no treatment at all for the 700,000 Americans—one third of them under age 65—hit by stroke each year.

This narrative is misleading on several fronts. It is not plausible that physicians could accurately conclude that Lucas "almost certainly would have died" without treatment. Nor is it true that "massive" strokes are likely to benefit from thrombolytic treatment (von Kummer *et al.* 1997). And of course, there is an unsupported implication that thrombolytics save lives.

3 This question is increasingly relevant in an age of terrorism. Public access to studies on biological or chemical warfare agents could enhance the informational resources of terrorists who want to use such weapons against civilians. For an interesting example, see Preston (2002).

4 This question has already received considerable attention from legal scholars (though not much from bioethicists). Good jurisprudence, like good journalism, should aim at the enlistment of unbiased expert testimony. Could we shift the impetus for obtaining "expert" testimony away from battling attorneys and toward judges or information

specialists employed by the court? Might the courts conscript specialists from a local roster—in a manner similar to the way they conscript jurists? Or could panels of non-industry-affiliated, non-research-oriented clinician-interpreters be utilized in the construction of legal standards of care? These or similar options provide fertile ground for discussion among ethicists concerned about the way we interpret scientific data.

5 I say "relatively new" because some work is already published or underway. Regarding the problem of thrombolytic therapy for acute stroke, see Furlan and Kanoti (1997) and Trotter (2002a).

6 Interestingly, the drug companies also receive money from the federal government to conduct drug trials—often through the agency of NIH officials who are on their payroll. See Willman (2003).

7 In federal funding, acquired immunodeficiency syndrome (AIDS), breast cancer, diabetes mellitus, and dementia all receive relatively generous support by almost any measurement standard, while research on chronic obstructive pulmonary disease, perinatal conditions, and peptic ulcer are relatively underfunded. See Gross *et al.* (1999).

8 *JAMA* devoted a whole issue to the peer-review process on July 15, 1998. The following articles are particularly interesting: Black *et al.* (1998) and Callaham *et al.* (1998).

9 See Hensley and Abboud, 2004; see also Anonymous, 2004. For another example of conflict over drug companies' role in suppressing data, see Burton (2000).

10 McLaughlin and Spencer report many instances of this tactic. Regarding a particularly juicy example, they write:

> This month [May 2004] at the American College of Obstetricians and Gynecologists annual meeting in Philadelphia, James Greenberg, an obstetrician gynecologist at Brigham and Women's Hospital in Boston, made a presentation about the benefits of cranberry juice cocktail for preventing urinary-tract infections. Dr. Greenberg is a paid consultant for *Ocean Spray Cranberries Inc*. Ocean Spray says it has long conducted research and marketed health information to consumers, but that in the past couple of years it has refocused energies on physicians.
>
> (2004)

11 An example of rigor in neutrality is a publication popular among physicians: *The Medical Letter*. I am not claiming that absolute neutrality is desirable or possible. But we should endeavor to distill out as much bias as possible—except, perhaps, for bias in the direction of medicine's fundamental values such as relieving suffering, curing disease, preventing untimely death, and so forth.

12 Philosopher Charles S. Peirce, for instance, has argued that effective researchers remain single mindedly focused on truth and largely detached from practical concerns. See Buchler (1955).

13 The external validity of a study is the applicability of study results to populations and practice settings other than those pertaining in the study. Several factors suggest that thrombolytic therapy might not work so well in settings exhibiting less experience, expertise, and equipment (Hankey 1997). First, it is essential to rule out intracranial hemorrhage (ICH), which causes about a third of strokes, in any patient considered for thrombolytics, since giving thrombolytics to ICH patients results in catastrophic, often fatal hemorrhage. ICH is ruled out by a negative CT scan of the brain. Studies show that nonacademic radiologists and neurologists are significantly less skilled than experts at detecting small hemorrhages on brain CT scans (Schriger *et al.* 1998). This difficulty is compounded in centers that lack the late generation CT scanners that were used in the NINDS trial. Second, even apart from the question of hemorrhage, the diagnosis of stroke is fraught with hazards and would presumably be less accurate in settings without highly experienced academic neurologists. Even neurologists unhurried by the three-hour treatment window sanctioned in the NINDS protocol are wrong almost 20 percent of the time when they diagnose stroke (Libman *et al.* 1995; Lille Stroke Program 1997). Third, it is unlikely that the strictures of the NINDS protocol would be applied as rigidly—even by excellent clinicians—as they were by researchers enacting the scientific protocol for

NINDS. A preview of the deleterious effects likely to pertain with widespread use of tPA for acute stroke in community hospitals is provided by Katzan and colleagues, who conducted a historical prospective cohort study of 3,948 patients diagnosed with acute ischemic stroke at 29 hospitals in the Cleveland area. Seventy patients received tPA. Of these, 11 patients (16 percent) had symptomatic brain hemorrhage and 6 of these patients died. Overall, mortality was 16 percent among patients receiving tPA and 5 percent in a matched subgroup of patients who did not receive tPA. In 50 percent of the cases, there were protocol violations, though there was no correlation between the protocol violations and the serious complications (Katzan *et al.* 2000).

14 One of the most common strategies for duping clinicians and the public is the publication and marketing of "equivalency studies" or "non-inferiority studies"—small studies that lack the power to show that one drug is superior to another, but which suggest that some new product is about equivalent to some established therapeutic mainstay. Frequently, the deck is loaded in such studies, for instance by administering low doses of the mainstay. In the end, the drug company usually claims that their new product is a preferable alternative to the (less expensive) mainstay because there may be fewer risks or side effects (limited experience in prescribing the drug means that less is known about the risks and side effects of new drugs—a fact that the drug companies manage to spin in their favor). See Smith (2003).

Bibliography

Abboud, L. (2003) "Expect a Food Fight as U.S. Revises Dietary Guidelines," *Wall Street Journal*, August 8, B1, B5.

Anonymous (2004) "When Drug Companies Hide Data," *New York Times*, June 6.

Baltic, S. (2001) "Conference Addresses Potential Flaws in Peer Review Process," *Journal of the National Cancer Institute*, 93(22): 1679–80.

Black, N., Van Rooyen, S., Godlee, F., Smith, R., and Evans, S. (1998) "What Makes a Good Reviewer and a Good Review for a General Medical Journal?," *Journal of American Medical Association*, 280(3): 231–33.

Bodenheimer, T. (2000) "Uneasy Alliance: Clinical Investigators and the Pharmaceutical Industry," *New England Journal of Medicine*, 342(20): 1539–43.

Buchler, J. (ed.) (1955) *Philosophical Writings of Peirce*, New York: Dover.

Burton, T.M. (2000) "Unfavorable Drug Study Sparks Battle over Publication of Results," *Wall Street Journal*, November 1, B1.

Callaham, M.L., Baxt, W.G., Waeckerle, J.F., and Wears, R.L. (1998) "Reliability of Editors' Subjective Quality Ratings of Peer Reviews of Manuscripts," *Journal of American Medical Association*, 280(3): 229–30.

Callahan, D. (1990) *What Kind of Life: The Limits of Medical Progress*, New York: Simon and Schuster.

Cantekin, E.I., McGuire, T.W., and Potter, R.L. (1990) "Biomedical Information, Peer Review, and Conflict of Interest as They Influence Public Health," *Journal of American Medical Association*, 263(10): 1427–30.

Caplan, L.R. (1997) "Stroke Thrombolysis—Growing Pains," *Mayo Clinic Proceedings*, 72: 1090–92.

Chan, A., Hrobjartsson, A., Haahr, M.T., Gotzsche, P.C., and Altman, D.G. (2004) "Empirical Evidence for Selective Reporting of Outcomes in Randomized Trials: Comparison of Protocols to Published Articles," *Journal of American Medical Association*, 291(20): 2457–65.

Choudry, N.K., Stelfox, H.T., and Detsky, A.S. (2002) "Relationships between Authors of Clinical Practice Guidelines and the Pharmaceutical Industry," *Journal of American Medical Association*, 287(5): 612–17.

DeAngelis, C.D., Fontanarosa, P.B., and Flanagin, A. (2001) "Reporting Financial Conflicts of Interest and Relationships between Investigators and Research Sponsors," *Journal of American Medical Association*, 286(1): 89–91.

Dewey, J. (1988) *The Later Works, 1925–1953: Volume 1: 1925: Experience and Nature*, J.A. Boydston (ed.), Carbondale and Edwardsville, IL: Southern Illinois University Press.

Donnan, G.A., Davis, S.M., Chambers, B.R., Gates, P.C., Hankey, G., McNeil, J.J., Rosen, D., Stewart-Wynne, E., and Tuck, R.R. (1996) "Streptokinase for Acute Ischemic Stroke With Relationship to Time of Administration," *Journal of American Medical Association*, 276(12): 961–66.

Evans, M. (1999) "Bioethics and the Newspapers," *Journal of Medicine and Philosophy*, 24: 164–80.

Frist, W.H. (2002) "Federal Funding for Biomedical Research: Commitment and Benefits," *Journal of American Medical Association*, 287(13): 1722–24.

Furlan, A.J. and Kanoti, G. (1997) "When Is Thrombolysis Justified in Patients with Acute Ischemic Stroke? A Bioethical Perspective," *Stroke*, 28: 214–18.

Goodman, K.W. (2003) *Ethics and Evidence-Based Medicine*, New York: Cambridge University Press.

Gross, C.P., Anderson, G.F., and Powe, N.R. (1999) "The Relation between Funding by the National Institutes of Health and the Burden of Disease," *New England Journal of Medicine*, 340(24): 1881–87.

Hacke, W., Kaste, M., Fieschi, C., Toni, D., Lesaffre, E., von Kummer, R., Boysen, G., Bluhmki, E., Hoxter, G., Mahagne, M., and Hennerici, M. (1995) "Intravenous Thrombolysis with Recombinant Tissue Plasminogen Activator for Acute Hemispheric Stroke: The European Cooperative Acute Stroke Study (ECASS)," *Journal of American Medical Association*, 274(13): 1017–25.

Hankey, G. (1997) "Thrombolytic Therapy in Acute Ischaemic Stroke: The Jury Needs More Evidence," *Medical Journal of Australia*, 166: 419–22.

Hensley, S. and Abboud, L. (2004) "Medical Research Has 'Black Hole'," *Wall Street Journal*, June 4, B3.

Hoffman, J.R. (2001) "Letter to the Editor," *Annals of Emergency Medicine*, 38(Annals Supplement on the American Heart Association Proceedings): 605.

Horrobin, D.F. (1990) "The Philosophical Basis of Peer Review and the Suppression of Innovation," *Journal of American Medical Association* 263(10): 1438–41.

Jorgensen, H.S., Nakayama, H., Kammersgaard, L.P., Raaschou, H.O., and Olsen, T.S. (1999) "Predicted Impact of Intravenous Thrombolysis on the Prognosis of General Population of Stroke Patients: Simulation Model," *British Medical Journal*, 319: 288–89.

Katzan, I.L., Furlan, A.J., Lloyd, L.E., Frank, J.I., Harper, D.L., Hinchey, J.A., Homel, J.P., Qu, A., and Silva, C.A. (2000) "Use of Tissue-Type Plasminogen Activator for Acute Ischemic Stroke: The Cleveland Area Experience," *Journal of American Medical Association*, 283(4): 1145–50.

Landis, D., Tarr, R.W., and Selman, W.R. (1997) "Thrombolysis for Acute Ischemic Stroke," *Neurosurgery Clinics of North America*, 8: 219–26.

Libman, R.B., Wirkowski, E., Alvir, J., and Rao, H. (1995) "Conditions that Mimic Stroke in the Emergency Department: Implication for Acute Stroke Trials," *Archives of Neurology*, 52(5): 1119–22.

Lille Stroke Program, Members of the (1997) "Misdiagnosis in 1,250 Consecutive Patients Admitted to an Acute Stroke Unit," *Cerebrovascular Diseases*, 7: 284–88.

McCormack, J. and Greenhalgh, T. (2000) "Seeing What You Want to See in Randomised Controlled Trials: Versions and Perversions of UKPDS Data," *British Medical Journal*, 320: 1720–23.

McLaughlin, K. and Spencer, J. (2004) "Take Two Grass-Fed Steaks and Call Me in the Morning," *Wall Street Journal*, May 25, D1.

Mills, A.E. and Spencer, E.M. (2003) "Evidence-Based Medicine: Why Clinical Ethicists Should Be Concerned," *HEC Forum*, 15(3): 231–44.

Misakian, A. and Bero, L.A. (1998) "Publication Bias and Research on Passive Smoking: Comparison of Published and Unpublished Studies," *Journal of American Medical Association*, 280(3): 250–53.

Moreno, J.D. (1995) *Deciding Together: Bioethics and Moral Consensus*, New York: Oxford University Press.

Multicenter Acute Stroke Trial, Europe Study Group (1996) "Thrombolytic Therapy with Streptokinase in Acute Ischemic Stroke," *New England Journal of Medicine*, 335(3): 145–50.

Multicentre Acute Stroke Trial, Italy (1995) "Randomised Controlled Trial of Streptokinas, Aspirin, and Combinations of Both in Treatment of Acute Ischaemic Stroke," *Lancet*, 346(8989): 1509–14.

National Institute of Neurological Disorders and Stroke, rt-PA Study Group (1995) "Tissue Plasminogen Activator for Acute Ischemic Stroke," *New England Journal of Medicine*, 333(24): 1581–87.

Peripheral and Central Nervous System Drugs Advisory Committee, Food and Drug Administration (1996) "Open Committee Discussion on Product License Application 96–0350 for Activase (alteplase), Genentech, for Management of Acute Stroke," Bethesda, MD: Food and Drug Administration.

Preston, R. (2002) *The Demon in the Freezer*, New York: Random House.

Rather, D. (1997) CBS Evening News, January 30.

Schriger, D.L., Kalafut, M., Starkman, S., Krueger, M., and Saver, J.L. (1998) "Cranial Computed Tomography Interpretation in Acute Stroke: Physician Accuracy in Determining Eligibility for Thrombolytic Therapy," *Journal of American Medical Association*, 279(16): 1293–97.

Schrof, J.M. (1999) "Stroke Busters: New Treatments in the Fight Against Brain Attacks," *US News and World Report*, March 15, 62–64, 68.

Smith, R. (2003) "Medical Journals and Pharmaceutical Companies: Uneasy Bedfellows," *British Medical Journal*, 326: 1202–05.

Stern, J.M. and Simes, R.J. (1998) "Publication Bias: Evidence of Delayed Publication in a Cohort Study of Clinical Research Projects," *British Medical Journal*, 315(7109): 640–45.

Trotter, G. (2002a) "Why Were the Benefits of tPA Exaggerated?" *Western Journal of Medicine*, 176: 194–97.

—— (2002b) "Moral Consensus in Bioethics: Illusive or Just Elusive?" *Cambridge Quarterly of Healthcare Ethics*, 11(1): 1–3.

von Kummer, R., Allen, K.L., Holle, R.L., Bozzao, L., Bastianello, S., Manelfe, C., Bluhmki, E., Ringelb, P., Meier, D.H., and Hacke, W. (1997) "Acute Stroke: Usefulness of Early CT Findings before Thrombolytic Therapy," *Radiology*, 205(2): 327–33.

Wazana, A. (2000) "Physicians and the Pharmaceutical Industry: Is a Gift Ever Really Just a Gift?" *Journal of American Medical Association*, 283(3): 373–80.

Willman, D. (2003) "Stealth Merger: Drug Companies and Government Medical Research," *Los Angeles Times*, December 7: A1.

Index